Treating Trauma and Traumatic Grief in Children and Adolescents

Treating Trauma and Traumatic Grief in Children and Adolescents

JUDITH A. COHEN
ANTHONY P. MANNARINO
ESTHER DEBLINGER

THE GUILFORD PRESS
New York   London

Library of Congress Cataloging-in-Publication Data
Cohen, Judith A.
  Treating trauma and traumatic grief in children and adolescents / Judith A. Cohen,
Anthony P. Mannarino, Esther Deblinger.
     p. cm.
  Includes bibliographical references and index.
  ISBN-13: 978-1-59385-308-2 (hard cover: alk. paper)
  ISBN-10: 1-59385-308-4 (hard cover: alk. paper)
  1. Post-traumatic stress disorder in children—Treatment.   2. Post-traumatic stress
disorder in adolescence—Treatment.   3. Psychic trauma in children—
Treatment.   4. Psychic trauma in adolescence—Treatment.   5. Grief in children—
Treatment.   6. Grief in adolescence—Treatment.   7. Cognitive therapy for
children.   8. Cognitive therapy for teenagers.   I. Mannarino, Anthony P.
II. Deblinger, Esther.   III. Title.
  RJ506.P55C66 2006
  618.92′8521—dc22

                                                              2006006987

About the Authors

Judith A. Cohen, MD, is a board certified child and adolescent psychiatrist, Medical Director of the Center for Traumatic Stress in Children and Adolescents at Allegheny General Hospital in Pittsburgh, and Professor of Psychiatry at Drexel University College of Medicine. With Anthony P. Mannarino and Esther Deblinger, she developed and tested trauma-focused cognitive-behavioral therapy (TF-CBT) for sexually abused and multiply traumatized children and their nonoffending parents over the past 20 years. Since 1983 Dr. Cohen has been funded by more than a dozen federally supported grants (including funding from the National Institute of Mental Health, the Substance Abuse and Mental Health Administration, and the U.S. Department of Justice) to conduct research related to the assessment and treatment of traumatized children. She has served on the Board of Directors of the American Professional Society on the Abuse of Children and received its Outstanding Professional Award in 2000. She is currently a member of the Board of Directors of the International Society for Traumatic Stress Studies, and is Associate Editor of the society's *Journal of Traumatic Stress,* as well as the first author of its published guidelines for treating childhood posttraumatic stress disorder. Dr. Cohen is the principal author of the *Practice Parameters for the Assessment and Treatment of Children and Adolescents with Posttraumatic Stress Disorder,* published by the American Academy of Child and Adolescent Psychiatry, which awarded her its 2004 Rieger Award for Scientific Achievement. She has also published and taught extensively on topics related to the assessment and treatment of childhood trauma.

Anthony P. Mannarino, PhD, is a licensed clinical psychologist, the Director of the Center for Traumatic Stress in Children and Adolescents at Allegheny General Hospital in Pittsburgh and Professor of Psychiatry at Drexel University College of Medicine. Dr. Mannarino has been a leader in the field of child traumatic stress for the past 25 years. He has been awarded numerous federal grants from the National Center on Child Abuse and Neglect and the National Institute of Mental Health to investigate the clinical course of traumatic stress symptoms in children and to develop effective treatment approaches for traumatized children and their families. He has received many honors for his work, including the Betty Elmer Outstanding Professional Award; the Most Outstanding Article Award for papers published in the journal *Child Maltreatment,* presented by the American Professional Society on the Abuse of Children (APSAC); the Model Program Award from the Substance Abuse and Mental Health Services Administration for "Cognitive Behavioral Therapy for Child Traumatic Stress"; and the Legacy Award from the Greater Pittsburgh Psychological Association. Dr. Mannarino recently completed a 2-year term as the president of APSAC and is president-elect of the Section on Child Maltreatment, Division 37, Child, Youth, and Family Services, of the American Psychological Association.

Esther Deblinger, PhD, is a licensed psychologist and Professor of Psychiatry at the University of Medicine and Dentistry of New Jersey (UMDNJ)–School of Osteopathic Medicine. She is also cofounder and codirector of the CARES (Child Abuse Research Education and Service) Institute, a member center of the National Child Traumatic Stress Network. Dr. Deblinger has been funded by the Foundation of UMDNJ, the National Center on Child Abuse and Neglect, and the National Institute of Mental Health to conduct extensive clinical research examining the mental health impact of child abuse and the treatment of posttraumatic stress disorder and other abuse-related difficulties. She has written numerous scientific articles and book chapters, as well as four books, including *Treating Sexually Abused Children and Their Nonoffending Parents: A Cognitive Behavioral Approach* (with Anne Hope Heflin) and the children's book *Let's Talk about Taking Care of You!: An Educational Book about Body Safety* (with Lori Stauffer). Dr. Deblinger is a frequent invited speaker at local, national, and international conferences; has served two terms on the Board of the American Professional Society on the Abuse of Children; and has been recognized by *Woman's Day* magazine and the New Jersey Office of the Child Advocate, and the Substance Abuse and Mental Health Administration, for her work in helping children overcome posttraumatic stress and other abuse-related difficulties. In addition to her administrative, research, and teaching responsibilities, Dr. Deblinger remains active as a clinician and supervisor.

Preface

This book grew out of our earlier treatment manuals and book (Cohen, Mannarino, & Deblinger, 2003; Cohen et al., 2001; Deblinger & Heflin, 1996), which described the use of trauma-focused cognitive-behavioral therapy (TF-CBT) for traumatized children, childhood traumatic grief, and children who experienced sexual abuse, respectively. While this book reflects our own research findings and incorporates important ideas from clinical research conducted by Edna Foa as well as others, a substantial amount has been an outgrowth of our recent collaborative efforts with community practitioners across the United States.

Over the past 8 years we have been fortunate to receive funding from the National Institute of Mental Health to conduct several treatment outcome studies at both of our centers: the Allegheny General Hospital Center for Traumatic Stress in Children and Adolescents and the CARES (Child Abuse Research Education and Service) Institute. One of these projects is now completed; the others are still ongoing. The completed study was conducted jointly at both centers and included more than 200 children and their parents. It was the first study to document the efficacy of TF-CBT for multiply traumatized children (Cohen, Deblinger, Mannarino, & Steer, 2004). In following up with these children a year after treatment was completed, we found that TF-CBT may be particularly helpful for children who have experienced multiple traumas or who have higher levels of depressive symptoms at the start of treatment (Deblinger, Mannarino, Cohen, & Steer, 2005). At the same time, the pilot studies for our childhood traumatic grief (CTG) model have produced very promising results (Cohen, Mannarino, & Knudsen, 2004; Cohen, Mannarino, & Staron, 2005). Given the strength of these findings, we believe that it is more important than ever for the TF-CBT model to be disseminated to community practitioners, since they are the therapists most likely to provide therapy to traumatized children.

Since the events of September 11, 2001, and the establishment of the National Child Traumatic Stress Initiative (www.nctsnet. org), funded by the Substance Abuse and Mental Health Services Administration (SAMHSA), the number of therapists requesting training in the TF-CBT and CTG treatment models has increased exponentially. These trainings have not been one-way experiences, however. While community-based providers were learning the TF-CBT model, we learned a great deal from them about how this model might be optimally implemented in frontline community settings, particularly with children from diverse cultural backgrounds and children with challenging clinical presentations and complex family situations. We have tried to incorporate much of what we learned into this book, and we thank all of the providers who shared their wisdom and expertise with us.

Until recently, many therapists have been averse to using treatment manuals, in part because they might have associated such manuals with rigid, uncreative types of therapeutic approaches. However, particularly since TF-CBT was recognized by SAMHSA as a "Model Program" for the treatment of childhood trauma and the prevention of substance abuse (www.modelprograms.samhsa.gov), we have been gratified by a deluge of requests for the TF-CBT and CTG treatment manuals.

The convergence of these three factors—emerging treatment findings regarding the efficacy of TF-CBT for multiply traumatized children and childhood traumatic grief, the revisions we were making to the treatment manuals based on valuable feedback from community treatment providers, and the increased demand for our treatment manuals—led to our decision to merge the previous three distinct manuals into this single book. We have divided the book into three sections: the first section introduces the concept of TF-CBT, while the second and third sections describe the specific trauma-focused and grief-focused components of this model, respectively. (As noted in the body of the book, however, it is commonly the case when treating traumatic grief in clinical practice that the trauma- and grief-focused components are intertwined to some degree.) We have also developed an easily remembered acronym for the TF-CBT components, PRACTICE, which is repeated frequently throughout the book. For each of the PRACTICE and grief-focused treatment components, we include both child and parent interventions, as well as cultural, developmental, and troubleshooting features.

We conclude the book with a brief section on treatment review and closure, followed by three appendices: Appendix 1 provides useful handouts and information sheets; Appendix 2 includes a list of resources for children, parents, and therapists; and Appendix 3 provides information on additional training for therapists.

We hope that this book meets the needs of therapists trying to learn about how to best implement the TF-CBT treatment model. However, as with any treatment model, it is rarely sufficient to simply read a book about how it works. To truly learn about this model, therapists would benefit by putting it into practice when treating traumatized children. If you are a treatment provider, in addition to reading the book, you might also consider supplementing it by taking the free TF-CBT online training course (available at www.musc.edu/tfcbt) or by attending one of the many TF-CBT trainings provided around the United States, and then try implementing the TF-CBT model in your clinical practice. Learning about the model from various sources and implementing it in your own practice are among the best ways to learn how TF-CBT can effectively treat trauma and traumatic grief in children. We welcome your comments, questions, and feedback about the TF-CBT model and hope to incorporate them in future revisions.

Acknowledgments

In developing this book over several years, we have benefited from the wisdom and clinical experience of many of our friends and colleagues across diverse disciplines. Our respective institutions, Allegheny General Hospital and the University of Medicine and Dentistry of New Jersey–School of Osteopathic Medicine, have provided very supportive environments in which to do our work. Moreover, our efforts in developing this treatment model would not have been possible without the support and assistance we have received from all our colleagues at each institution. The therapists and supervisors who have implemented the trauma-focused cognitive-behavioral therapy model in our clinics and treatment studies have provided particularly valuable insights and creative ideas, and we thank them greatly for their many contributions.

We would also like to thank the funding agencies that have supported us in developing and testing this treatment model: the National Center on Child Abuse and Neglect (NCCAN, which is now the Office on Child Abuse and Neglect; OCAN), the National Institute of Mental Health (NIMH), the Substance Abuse and Mental Health Services Administration (SAMHSA), the Jewish Healthcare Foundation of Pittsburgh, the Staunton Farm Foundation of Pittsburgh, and the Foundation of the University of Medicine and Dentistry of New Jersey.

We would also like to thank our colleagues in the National Child Traumatic Stress Network (NCTSN), a collection of trauma treatment programs across the United States, funded by SAMHSA, as well as other professionals in the fields of child abuse and child trauma who have provided ongoing constructive suggestions for revising this book to be more responsive to the needs of community therapists working with traumatized children. These friends and colleagues, too numerous to mention by name, include those we have known for over 20 years as well as those we have met more recently. We have benefited from their steadfast professional and personal support and encouragement throughout the development and testing of this treatment approach. We also acknowledge the therapists and directors of the Columbia University-coordinated Child and Adolescent Trauma Treatment Services (CATS) program and the National Crime Victims Research and Treatment Center at the Medical University of South Carolina, who have provided valuable insights regarding the role of culture in implementing this model.

Developing, revising, and testing the child traumatic grief treatment components described in this book were undertaken, in part, through the support of the NCTSN's Child Traumatic Grief Work Group. Our colleagues at the Allegheny General Hospital Center for Traumatic Stress in Children and Adolescents, Tamra Greenberg, Susan Padlo, Carrie Seslow, and Karen Stubenbort, were particularly instrumental in conceptualizing earlier versions of these child traumatic grief components, and we thank them for their important contributions.

We are deeply grateful to Ann Marie Kotlik, who has worked closely and loyally with us for 20 years. Her skillful dedication has contributed enormously to this book, and we thank her for this and her countless other important contributions to our program.

We are most appreciative of the patience, love, and support we have each received from our families.

Finally, we thank the many parents and children who, at very difficult times in their lives, have entrusted themselves in our care. We feel privileged to have had the opportunity to learn from them. They have reinforced for us the central importance of the child–parent bond and the healing power of this connection.

We dedicate this book to all of the children with whom we have worked, and to our own children.

Contents

PART I

TRAUMA-FOCUSED COGNITIVE-BEHAVIORAL THERAPY

CHAPTER 1

The Impact of Trauma and Grief on Children and Families

WHAT CONSTITUTES CHILDHOOD TRAUMA?

Many children[1] experience stressful events as they are growing up. They are faced with painful situations, such as parental divorce or the death of a beloved elderly relative, which may be difficult and stressful to varying degrees. Yet these experiences would not usually be considered traumatic, a qualitatively different experience. Features that distinguish traumatic events include the following: sudden or unexpected events; the shocking nature of such events; death or threat to life or bodily integrity; and/or the subjective feeling of intense terror, horror, or helplessness (American Psychiatric Association [APA], 2000, p. 463). Some examples include child physical or sexual abuse; witnessing or being the direct victim of domestic, community, or school violence; severe motor vehicle and other accidents; potentially life-threatening illnesses, such as cancer, burns, or organ transplantation; natural and human-made disasters; sudden death of a parent, sibling, or peer; and exposure to war, terrorism, or refugee conditions. Even after experiencing such traumatic events, many children are resilient and do not develop enduring trauma symptoms. Several factors, including developmental level, inherent or learned resiliency, and external sources of support, may influence which children will develop difficulties.

A child's response to a traumatic event will be mediated by his/her age and developmental level. For example, it appears that for short-lived

[1]Throughout this book, the term *children* is used to refer to children and adolescents.

3

traumas, younger children are more dependent on their parents' reaction to that trauma than older children (regardless of how great their exposure); if their parents cope well, most younger children do not develop serious or long-lasting trauma symptoms (Laor, Wolmer, & Cohen, 2001). Yet ongoing traumas that start early in life have the potential to dramatically alter the trajectory of young children's development more than chronic traumas that begin later in adolescence. Thus, in some traumatic circumstances, younger age may be protective whereas in other circumstances, it may confer greater risk.

Similarly, the impact of an identical stressor may vary considerably from child to child depending on each child's inherent resiliency, learned coping mechanisms, and external sources of physical, emotional, and social support. Even stressors that would universally be considered traumatic (e.g., witnessing multiple murders or being the victim of rape) are experienced as being less traumatic by some children than by others. We have often observed this marked range of responses to identical traumas among siblings in the same family exposed to the same horrific events. For example, in one case of longstanding domestic violence, the father shot the mother in front of the children, killed the youngest son, and then killed himself. All of the surviving children were present when this occurred. However, all three children had markedly different responses. The youngest surviving child, a 7-year-old girl, had severe symptoms of posttraumatic stress disorder (PTSD); the 14-year-old son had no apparent PTSD or depressive symptoms but had serious aggression problems that required inpatient hospitalization; the 12-year-old daughter had only moderate depressive symptoms and focused on caring for and comforting her younger sister. Thus the experience of trauma depends not only upon exposure to a traumatic event but also on the individual child's response to that event

This response variation occurs, in part, because children have unique ways of understanding traumatic events, making meaning of these events in relation to themselves, accessing familial and other forms of support, coping with the psychological and physiological stress associated with these events, and integrating these events into their larger sense of self. The treatment approach described in this book offers interventions to optimize each of these steps in the process of helping children cope with traumatic events and can be tailored to address the needs of individual children.

The treatment model described in this book, trauma-focused cognitive-behavioral therapy (TF-CBT), was developed for children who have been traumatized, as indicated by the symptoms described in the next section. The model may not be appropriate for children without these symptoms. Specifically, children who do not have symptoms of PTSD, depression, or anxiety will likely not need all of the components covered in this treatment approach. For example, a child who has few hyperarousal and avoidance symptoms, little anxiety, and no depression related to the traumatic experience will most likely have little need to create a trauma narrative in therapy; such a child will likely be easily able to talk about his trauma experiences early in treatment with a minimum of encouragement. Such a child might benefit from an attenuated version of TF-CBT that would include, for example, psychoeducation, relaxation training, affective modulation, and perhaps some cognitive-processing components. This is not to say that directly discussing what happened would have no value for such children but only that they may not need to spend a great deal of time in therapy doing so.

This book also describes treatment for children who have experienced traumatic grief, that is, the loss of a loved one under traumatic circumstances. When trauma symptoms occur in the context of the death of a loved one, the child and parent not only have to address their trauma symptoms but also cope with the fact that these trauma symptoms often interfere with, and impinge on, their ability to negotiate typical grieving processes. Left unaddressed, this added factor may leave children with unresolved grief for years to come. The traumatic grief treatment approach described in this book integrates trauma- and grief-focused components in a sequential manner, such that once trauma symptoms have abated, the child and parent are able to begin the grieving process. The trauma-focused treatment components are described in Part II of this book, while the grief-focused treatment components are described in Part III. Children who have serious levels of dysfunction in multiple domains (as described below) in addition to trauma symptoms may also need other types of interventions or stabilization strategies.

Finally, there are circumstances in which children endure highly stressful events but are able to adjust well with support and guidance from caregivers as well as other resources in their communities. Unfortunately, however, a significant proportion of children who have suffered trauma also experience emotional and behavioral symptoms that persist into adolescence and adulthood.

WHAT ARE TRAUMA SYMPTOMS?

The term *trauma symptoms*, as used in this book, refers to behavioral, cognitive, physical, and/or emotional difficulties that are directly related to the traumatic experience. These typically correspond to symptoms of

PTSD, but also encompass other depressive, anxiety, or behavioral symptoms, including self-injury, substance abuse, impaired interpersonal trust, and affective instability. Children with trauma symptoms may experience a profound change in the way they see themselves, the world, and/or other people as a result of their exposure to one or more traumatic events. There is growing evidence that many of these children also experience psychobiological changes that may contribute to the development and maintenance of these psychological symptoms. We have divided these symptoms into several general categories: *affective, behavioral, cognitive, complex PTSD,* and *psychobiological* trauma symptoms. As will become evident, these divisions are somewhat arbitrary in that these areas of difficulty overlap and interact continuously.

Affective Trauma Symptoms

Common *affective* trauma symptoms include fear, depression, anger, and affective dysregulation (i.e., frequent mood changes and/or difficulty tolerating negative affective states). *Fear* is both an instinctive and learned reaction to frightening situations. Children often instinctively experience fear in life-threatening situations; the autonomic nervous system responds to this perceived danger by releasing large amounts of adrenergic neurotransmitters, which can further reinforce anxiety. Fearful memories are also encoded in the brain differently than those from nontraumatic memories. Some children will subsequently experience the same physiological and psychological fear reactions when exposed to reminders of the traumatic event (e.g., a child who was in a serious car accident, which may have included a fatality, may become terrified whenever he/she rides past the site of the accident). This fear response can become generalized so that people, places, things, or situations that are inherently innocuous but that remind the child of the traumatic event will cause the same level of fear as the original trauma (e.g., this child might experience intense fear when riding in any car). The intrusion of fearful memories is a hallmark of PTSD; children may have intrusive, frightening thoughts during the day or scary dreams at night. In younger children the content of these scary dreams may not be related to the traumatic event in an obvious way, but may be about other frightening things; the development of new fears (with no apparent relationship to the trauma other than temporal proximity) may be a PTSD symptom in very young children (Scheeringa, Zeanah, Myers, & Putnam, 2003).

In addition to specific fears, *general anxiety* may develop due to the sudden, unexpected, terrifying nature of the trauma. This may lead children to feel generally unsafe and hypervigilant, on guard to protect themselves from being "taken by surprise the next time." A sense of impending doom (the "sword of Damocles" hanging over their heads) can impinge on children's ability to engage in developmentally appropriate tasks and contribute to their taking on responsibilities well beyond a maturity level typical for their age. General anxiety can result in the "parentification" of a child or contribute to a child's effort to be "perfect" to ward off potential threats in the future. A constant vigilance for possible omens of future threats and other anxiety-driven behaviors can also take hold. All of these behaviors interfere with healthy adjustment and can lead to the development of comorbid generalized anxiety disorder as well as other comorbidities.

Children may experience *depressive feelings* after a trauma, which may arise in response to an abrupt loss of trust in other people and the world (e.g., loss of innocence, trust, faith, or hope in the future). Many traumatized children experience more concrete losses; for example, a child who is shot or hit by a car may temporarily or permanently experience a loss of function or damaged appearance of body parts. A child who is sexually abused may lose his/her "virginity" or experience other painful genital injuries. A fire or natural disaster may result in children's loss of personal belongings, their homes, or even the lives of loved ones. Children's developmentally normal egocentric view of the world may lead to self-blame for the traumatic event, which in turn may lead to depressive symptoms that include guilt, shame, diminished self-esteem, feelings of worthlessness, and even suicidality. Negative self-image—an important issue for many traumatized children—can contribute to maladaptive choices in peers and romantic partners and self-destructive behaviors such as substance abuse, cutting, unsafe sexual practices, and suicide attempts, all of which are strongly associated with a history of child abuse or other traumas. The bottom line: Depressive disorders often occur in combination with PTSD symptoms.

Anger may result from the child's awareness that the traumatic event was unfair, that is, that he/she didn't do anything bad enough to "deserve" the trauma. Other children, particularly those experiencing physical abuse or bullying, may develop anger as they observe the behavior of caretakers or others who cope inappropriately with difficulties or frustrations. Children experiencing domestic violence may develop "traumatic bonding" (Bancroft & Silverman, 2002, pp. 39–41), in which they realize that their safety depends on aligning themselves with the abuser (discussed in more detail later in the chapter). Anger in traumatized children may take the form of noncompliant behavior, unpredictable rages or tantrums, or physical aggression toward property or other people. Children who have experienced sexual abuse may also engage in sexual aggression toward others. It is important to keep in mind that some traumatized children may have had anger or behavioral problems that predated, and are unrelated to, the traumatic events.

Severely or chronically traumatized children may become highly *sensitive* and *overreactive* to behaviors or situations that they associate with previous traumas. For example, one study indicated that children who have been physically abused perceive angry faces (a presumed trauma cue for children who have been physically abused) much more readily than nonphysically abused children (Pine et al., 2005). Chronically maltreated children may develop a dysfunctional degree of hypersensitivity to perceived rejection because parental or other rejection in their past experience was associated with, and served as an early warning signal for, abusive or other traumatic acts. Severely traumatized children often display *affective dysregulation*, that is, sudden changes in affective state and/or difficulty coping with negative affective states. Anecdotally, affective dysregulation seems to occur more commonly in children who have experienced interpersonal violence, such as child abuse or domestic violence, than in children who have experienced a single, nonintentional traumatic event. Chronically traumatized children often have not received a nurturing, soothing response from others during or immediately following the traumatization; in contrast, many of these children have experienced their fear, sadness, or anger being invalidated, ignored, or responded to negatively by the perpetrator and/or others. For example, a child who witnesses domestic violence may be told to "shut up" not only by the perpetrating parent, but also by the victimized parent (who is afraid of further angering the batterer). Thus neither parent in this situation may acknowledge the child's legitimate emotions, or provide comfort and soothing, or model appropriate affective modulation. Chronically traumatized children also have been found to have neurobiological alterations, including chronic elevation of stress hormones and adrenergic neurotransmitters such as epinephrine (adrenaline), that would tend to make affective modulation more difficult (DeBellis et al., 1999). Thus there may be both psychological and neurobiological components to affective dysregulation in chronically traumatized children.

Behavioral Trauma Symptoms

In an attempt to avoid painful feelings, children may develop behaviors that, although meant to protect them from pain, may lead to more difficulties. *Avoidance* of trauma reminders is a hallmark of PTSD. In order to escape overwhelming negative feelings, children may try to avoid any thoughts, people, places, or situations that remind them of their traumatic experiences. If these reminders extensively generalize, significant constriction of developmentally appropriate activities may occur. For example, a child who was sexually abused at night may become generally fearful at night and avoid being in unfamiliar settings at night, such as sleepovers at friends' homes. An adolescent whose brother was hit by a car might refuse to learn to drive, or a child who was beaten up on the playground may avoid going to school. In many instances, it is impossible for children to avoid all trauma reminders. For example, for a child who witnessed ongoing domestic violence, both parents may be trauma reminders; for a child experiencing pervasive ongoing community violence, his/her whole neighborhood may become a trauma trigger. For children whose trauma reminders have become generalized to the point of being ubiquitous, avoidance is rarely a successful long-term management strategy. When avoidance is unsuccessful in protecting children from overwhelming negative emotions, they may develop emotional *numbing*, or in more severe cases, *dissociation*. Recent debates have centered around the issue of whether avoidance (volitional behavioral symptoms) and numbing (automatic, uncontrollable responses) should, in fact, be considered two separate PTSD clusters because numbing is not under a person's behavioral control (Asmundson, Stapleton, & Taylor, 2004).

Trauma-related behaviors may also develop in response to modeling or traumatic bonding (Bancroft & Silverman, 2002). Modeling occurs when children who grow up in abusive or violent homes and communities have many opportunities to observe and learn *maladaptive behaviors* and coping strategies. They may also see those behaviors being rewarded repeatedly. For example, a child who experiences physical abuse and domestic violence may erroneously conclude that anger and abuse are accepted ways of coping with frustration. If this child also sees the abusive parent as having control over the family's activities, emotional tone, finances, etc., whereas the battered parent is repeatedly injured and powerless, he/she may conclude that battering is an acceptable and even advantageous behavior. As another example, *sexualized behaviors* are modeled during sexual abuse; if the sexually abused child learns that these behaviors are rewarding (either through the power they confer to the abuser over the abused or because they are physically stimulating), this child may develop ongoing sexualized behaviors. A final example is that of a community bully or drug dealer. If such people are perceived as powerful and admired by others, as being rewarded for their bullying, violent, or illegal behaviors, then children may conclude that these behaviors are desirable and therefore copy them, unless alternative rewarding models are present in their immediate environment.

Traumatic bonding involves both modeling of inappropriate behaviors and maladaptive attachment dynamics. It also involves acceptance of inaccurate explanations for inappropriate behaviors. It has been described in the psychoanalytic literature as identification with the aggressor and in law enforcement as the Stockholm syndrome. When children are under the control of a violent or aggressive parent and the other parent is ineffectual at self- or child protection, their natural needs for parental attachment and affiliation become distorted and conflicted. In this situation, it is difficult to remain equally affiliated with both parents without experiencing great confusion and conflict. Often such children both fear and love the abusive parent, and may have experienced abuse personally if they attempted to defend the abused parent. Such children may bond with the violent parent out of self-preservation. To manage the guilt and cognitive dissonance associated with turning against the victimized parent, these children may adopt the violent parent's views, attitudes, and behaviors toward the victimized parent and become abusive or violent themselves. For example, a parent who batters his or her spouse may blame the battering behavior on the battered parent (e.g., "If you had dinner ready on time, this never would have happened"), and the child who is traumatically bonded may display anger or aggression toward the battered parent for "making" the batterer perpetrate this episode of battering. Thus it is clear that modeling and traumatic bonding can contribute to aggressive behaviors in traumatized children.

Other problematic behaviors that may be trauma related often develop in traumatized children. For example, these children may avoid healthy age-appropriate peer interactions, preferring to associate with peers who have emotional and/or behavioral problems. These choices may be related to the negative self-image that many traumatized children develop, as discussed above; because of fear of rejection by "normal" peers; and/or because for children living with ongoing interpersonal maltreatment, associating with troubled peers may seem more familiar or comfortable. As noted above, many traumatized children develop *anger* that is manifested through oppositional, aggressive, or destructive behaviors. Traumatized children are also at greater risk for *substance abuse*, which may be used as a strategy for avoiding trauma reminders, a way of coping with negative self-image, or may arise as a result of associating with other troubled children. *Self-injury*, such as cutting, burning, or other forms of self-mutilation, and suicidal behaviors are also associated with childhood trauma. Some self-injurious youth describe these as methods for reversing the numbness that they feel. For example, one youth said, "When I hurt from cutting myself, it's the only time I know that I am real." Others may be seeking attention which they feel unable to gain in more adaptive ways; still others may be reacting to the despair and unbearable pain they feel by truly trying to harm themselves. Some youth describe the cutting behavior as a means of managing anxiety. The dangerousness of some children's behaviors will warrant a treatment approach that first focuses on diminishing these behaviors and assuring safety rather than addressing the underlying traumatic etiology of the behaviors.

Cognitive Trauma Symptoms

Childhood trauma can also distort children's cognitions (thoughts) about themselves, the perpetrator(s) of trauma, other people, the social contract, and the world. Following a traumatic event, children will typically search for an explanation for why something so terrible has happened to them or their loved ones. If no rational explanation is found, children may develop *irrational beliefs* about causation in order to gain some sense of control or predictability. In our experience the most common irrational belief involves children blaming themselves, either by taking responsibility for the event itself ("He sexually abused me because of how I dressed") or for not foreseeing and avoiding the event (e.g., "I should have known Dad would be in a bad mood—why didn't I warn Mom to leave the house so he wouldn't have beaten her up?"; "I should have stopped my brother from going to school today so he wouldn't have gotten shot on the way home"). Alternatively, although not blaming themselves directly for the traumatic event, children may come to believe that they are bad, shameful, or otherwise lacking in some way that "justifies" bad things happening to them (e.g., "There must be something wrong with me for this to have happened to me"). In this manner the world remains fair, predictable, and makes sense; it is only *they* who are deserving of bad fortune. Children exposed to ongoing interpersonal trauma (child abuse or neglect, domestic violence) seem particularly prone to these types of cognitions, perhaps because these acts are intentional, personally directed, and typically perpetrated by parents or other adults who would ordinarily be expected to protect rather than harm children. Developing realistic cognitions of responsibility (i.e., blaming the perpetrator) may be extremely difficult and painful for these children.

Other cognitive distortions may develop in relation to other people (i.e., nonperpetrators). Children may generalize their experience of betrayal by one person to mean that *no one* is trustworthy. This belief can lead to difficulties in peer relationships or in the child's attachment to the nonoffending parent and other adults, which may further contribute to the child's impaired self-image (i.e., the child undermines these relationships, then attributes the disappointment to his/her own personal failings). Alternatively, children may respond to a betrayal of trust by repeatedly trying to "correct" or reverse their experience by seeking out inappropriately close relationships with peers or adults who may or may not be safe in this regard. This strategy often leads to additional painful experiences in the form of repeated maltreatment or through rejection of the child's inappropriate or unwarranted expectations for closeness. Traumatized children may also develop cognitions that contribute to their loss of faith in justice, God, or a benign future. This line of thinking can lead to behavioral choices that become "self-fulfilling prophecies." For example, a teen who lost his older brother and several friends to community violence developed the belief that he was not going to live to see his 20th birthday. As a result, he began to use drugs, joined a gang, and dropped out of school. These behaviors greatly diminished his chances of experiencing a positive future and put him at increased risk for trauma. His own negative expectations or "prophecy" of self-failure led to the very failure he feared.

In some cases children have accurate cognitions that are not helpful because they are not contextualized or they focus only on the negative aspects of situations. For example, the cognition "You never know who will sexually abuse you" might be true in a given environment, but equally true is the alternative cognition, "Most men do not sexually abuse children." It is clear that the first thought is likely to promote fear and avoidance, whereas the second, equally accurate thought is more reassuring and hopeful. Traumatized children often focus on inaccurate and/or unhelpful cognitions that reinforce their negative expectations of others and their destructive self-views. These cognitive symptoms contribute significantly to the maintenance of PTSD, other forms of anxiety, and depressive and behavioral difficulties.

"Complex PTSD"

In the face of repeated or ongoing traumatic life events, some children (particularly adolescents) may develop pervasive difficulties in multiple, important domains, including affective regulation, interpersonal relationships, self-esteem and self-efficacy, academic and vocational functioning, and maintenance of personal safety. Such children may present with a constellation of problems that includes severe mood instability or irritability, highly conflicted relationships and difficulty maintaining friendships, poor self-esteem and lack of interpersonal trust, academic difficulties (poor grades, truancy, dropping out of school or engaging in problematic behaviors in the school setting), and self-injurious behaviors (including substance abuse). This constellation of difficulties has sometimes been referred to as complex PTSD. To our knowledge, only one controlled treatment trial has been completed (Najavits, 1998) and another initiated (Cloitre, Davis, & Mirvis, 2002) for such youth; however, findings are not yet available from these studies. These studies have incorporated TF-CBT components along with initial intensive relationship-building and safety-enhancing components (Najavits, 2002). Other groups have described promising treatments for chronically traumatized teens, but these treatments have not yet been principally tested (DeRosa, 2004). Although our treatment studies have included a few such youth, we have not systematically evaluated the efficacy of TF-CBT for this population of chronically traumatized adolescents. In our multisite study, which included multiply traumatized children from poor, multiproblem families (Cohen, Deblinger, Mannarino, & Steer, 2004), the chronically traumatized youth responded well to the TF-CBT treatment approach. In fact, the findings of follow-up analyses seem to suggest that children reporting multiple traumas and higher levels of depression at pretreatment showed greater treatment responsiveness to TF-CBT than to a less structured client-centered approach (Deblinger, Mannarino, Cohen, & Steer, 2005).

Our view is that trauma effects occur along a continuum, from *no* or *minimally detectable* difficulties to *overwhelming problems* in multiple areas of functioning. Although exposure to past trauma is a risk factor for more severe psychopathology upon retraumatization (Pine & Cohen, 2002), many children and adolescents show remarkable resilience even in the face of severe and repeated trauma. Other factors have been shown to mediate the impact of trauma on children, including parental support and level of distress as well as each child's trauma-related attributions and perceptions (Cohen & Mannarino, 1996b, 2000; Deblinger, Steer, & Lippmann, 1999; Kliewer, Murrelle, Mejia, Torresde, & Angold, 2001; Laor et al., 2001). Although we cannot control a child's past trauma exposure, our TF-CBT model does attempt to exert an impact on parents' functioning and children's trauma-related cognitions in a manner that reduces the likelihood of more severe and long-lasting difficulties. We recognize that this treatment approach may be insufficient for some traumatized children or adolescents; however, we believe that its major components have application for the majority of this population.

The Psychobiological Impact of Trauma

Children's brains and bodies are integrally involved in the development and manifestation of emotions, cognitive processes, and behaviors. It is important to understand that everything a person does, thinks, or feels is associated with some brain activity, however transient or inconsequential. Thus it is not surprising that trauma events have the potential to alter brain functioning. When these changes in brain functioning are maintained over a long period (in some cases long after the traumatic events have ended), they may contribute to the maintenance of many of the trauma symptoms described earlier. In some cases, these chronic functional alterations may also contribute to *structural* changes in the brain.

Many people are unaware of the fact that the physical structure of the brain is dynamic—which means that, within limits, brain structure is interactive with brain functioning. For example, the number of receptors in the brain for different neurotransmitters can be increased or decreased in response to many factors, including stress. Stress is known to change neurotransmitter and hormonal activity both in the brain and in other parts of the body (e.g., adrenal glands), which in turn produce physiological responses such as increased heart rate, respirations, and blood pressure, diversion of blood flow to skeletal muscles, and increased alertness. Childhood trauma, and PTSD in particular, are associated with chronic changes in these areas of physiology; that is, traumatized children may have higher resting pulse rates and blood pressure, greater physical tension, and hypervigilance. Other alterations in brain function and structure have been documented in traumatized children, particularly those who have experienced interpersonal traumas such as child abuse or domestic violence. For example, in one study, children who had a history of sexual abuse, physical abuse, or exposure to domestic violence were found to have smaller intracranial volume (brain size), lower IQs, poorer grades, smaller corpus collosi (the part of the brain that connects the right and left hemispheres), and higher dissociation scores than children who did not have such trauma histories. Furthermore, the severity of these changes was correlated with the length of time the maltreatment had occurred (DeBellis et al., 1999).

Given that the function and structure of the brain are interactive with our life experiences, thoughts, feelings, and behaviors, it would make sense that a return to more adaptive psychological functioning would be associated with corresponding normalization of brain function and, perhaps, structure. This line of thinking suggests that therapeutic (or other) interventions that result in reregulation of children's emotional, cognitive, and behavioral functioning can minimize or reverse the adverse impact of trauma on their brains and bodies.

Some professionals believe that only certain types of therapeutic activities can access pathways for brain changes (e.g., directed eye movements or body therapy techniques), and that "talking" therapies that do not include specified, physical activities cannot create meaningful brain or bodily changes in traumatized children. We suggest that it is possible to restore adaptive psychobiological functioning in a variety of ways, including through the use of psychotherapeutic components incorporated in the TF-CBT model. We are currently collaborating with the National Institute of Mental Health and other colleagues to evaluate the psychobiological impact of providing TF-CBT to traumatized children, and we welcome hearing the results of studies using other therapies for these children. However, we believe that even if certain traumagenic functional or structural brain changes do not respond to psychotherapy, this does not diminish the value of psychotherapy in reducing children's symptoms and improving their adaptive functioning and quality of life.

THE IMPACT OF TRAUMATIC GRIEF ON CHILDREN

When children lose a loved one to an unexpected, violent, or gory death, or when they are exposed to graphic details such as blood, mutilated or missing body parts, or being the first person to discover the body of the loved one, they may develop a condition known as childhood traumatic grief (CTG). (See p. 17 for a more detailed discussion of CTG.) Examples include death due to interpersonal violence (community, domestic, or school settings), motor vehicle or other accidents, suicide of a family member or peer, natural disasters, or acts of terrorism. In these cases children are dealing with both trauma and loss, and they need the components described in Part II of this book as well as the additional treatment components that allow them to begin the process of grieving the death of a loved one presented in Part III.

First, it may be helpful to define some terms related to grief, bereavement, and loss.

Uncomplicated grief refers to the normal process of grieving for the loss of an important relationship. This condition resembles the diagnosis of major depressive disorder (MDD) in several ways, and MDD is typically not diagnosed in the first 2 months after the death of a loved one, unless the bereaved person has

> 1) guilt about things other than actions taken or not taken by the survivor at the time of death; 2) thoughts of death other than the survivor feeling that he or she would be better off dead or should have died with the deceased person; 3) morbid preoccupation with worthlessness; 4) marked psychomotor retardation; 5) prolonged or marked functional impairment; and 6) hallucinatory experiences other than thinking that he or she hears the voice of, or transiently sees the image of, the deceased person. (APA, 2000, p. 741)

Although early writings suggested that there were standard "stages" of grieving, as described by Kübler-Ross and others, more recent authors have contested this format (Simpson, 1997). There is also great variability in how long it takes people to complete "normal" grieving. Typical tasks of uncomplicated grief for children have been described by Worden (1996) and Wolfelt (1991). These include the following tasks:

- Experiencing the deep pain associated with the loss of the loved one.
- Accepting the permanence of the loss (this will vary somewhat according to the developmental level of the child).
- Reminiscing about the deceased loved one and accepting the totality of the loved one—the good and the bad.
- Converting the relationship from one of interaction to one of memory.
- Incorporating important aspects of the loved one into the child's own self-identity.
- Committing to new relationships.
- Reestablishing a healthy developmental trajectory.

Complicated grief refers to grief accompanied by symptoms of separation distress and trauma (Prigerson, Shear, & Jacobs, 1999; Prigerson et al., 1997), in reference to adults, this term has been used interchangeably with the term "traumatic grief" (Prigerson et al., 1997). Complicated grief in adults typically occurs following a death that would not objectively be considered as "traumatic" (i.e., not resulting from an unanticipated, horrifying event) and requires that the person experience (1) extreme levels of three of the four "separation distress" symptoms (intrusive thoughts about the deceased; yearning for the deceased; searching for the deceased; and excessive loneliness since the death), as well as (2) extreme levels of four of the eight "traumatic distress" symptoms (purposelessness about the future; numbness, detachment, or absence of emotional responsiveness; difficulty believing or acknowledging the death; feeling that life is empty or meaningless; feeling that part of oneself has died; shattered world view; assuming symptoms of harmful behaviors of the deceased person; excessive irritability, bitterness, or anger related to the death) (Prigerson & Jacobs, 2001). Additionally, these symptoms must have lasted at least 6 months (criterion C) and lead to significant functional impairment (criterion D). Complicated grief can be measured by the Inventory of Complicated Grief (ICG; Prigerson et al., 1995) and is associated with increased risk of psychiatric comorbidity and physical illness in adults.

The term *traumatic grief* has been used somewhat variably in the child literature. In this book *childhood traumatic grief* (CTG) refers to a condition in which both unresolved grief and PTSD symptoms are present, often accompanied by depressive symptoms as well. The unresolved grief symptoms are similar to those described in adult complicated grief (i.e., yearning and searching for the deceased and difficulty in accepting the death). The PTSD symptoms include intrusive/preoccupying thoughts; dreams or memories about the traumatic death and/or the deceased; avoidance of reminders of the deceased; and/or the trauma reminders related to the death; emotional numbness or detachment; and hyperarousal symptoms, including anger or bitterness related to the death (Brown & Goodman, 2005; Layne, Saltzman, Savjak, & Pynoos, 1999; Nader, 1997; Melham et al., 2004; Pynoos, 1992; Rando, 1996).

WHY DISTINGUISH CTG
FROM OTHER FORMS OF GRIEF?

Even when it involves the loss of a parent, uncomplicated grief in childhood does not appear to place children at increased risk for ongoing mental illness, provided that they experience adequate parenting following the death (Harrington & Harrison, 1999). However, the presence of significant childhood PTSD symptoms place children at risk for developing other serious psychiatric conditions, including depression, substance abuse, and borderline personality disorder, which may last into adulthood and beyond (American Academy of Child and Adolescent Psychiatry [AACAP], 1998). We believe that when PTSD symptoms are accompanied by unresolved grief symptoms, it may be insufficient to provide either trauma- or grief-focused interventions alone. Therefore, it may be important to identify those children with CTG and provide them with combined trauma- and grief-focused treatment so that they will not have long-lasting PTSD symptoms and can at last move forward in beginning to resolve the typical tasks of grieving.

PHASE-ORIENTED TREATMENT

Based on the work of many authors as well as our clinical experience, it appears that when trauma and grief symptoms are both present, it is advisable, and often essential, to address and at least partially resolve the trauma issues before the grief issues can be successfully addressed (Nader, 1997; Rando, 1996; Layne et al., 1999). This principle may be particularly applicable for certain traumatic reminders or obsessions; for example, when a child is fixated on the most horrifying aspects of the dead body or does not have accurate information on how the person died and repeatedly imagines "worst-case" scenarios. Often in such children even positive memories of the deceased (an important aspect of negotiating the grief process) segue into traumatic reminders—that is, the child can't think of the deceased without remembering the terrifying details of the death. Additionally, children who have avoidance symptoms may be so detached from their feelings that they are unable to experience their grief. For these reasons, some trauma-focused interventions are typically utilized in the beginning phase of treating CTG, with grief issues addressed later in treatment. However, individual children progress at their own pace and on their own path. Some children will resolve most or all trauma symptoms before moving on to grief issues, but many children will need to intersperse grief and trauma work, according to which issues are most problematic at different times. Thus the trauma and grief phases of treatment may be interwoven, as clinically indicated.

External factors may also influence the phasing of treatment. For example, investigation, media attention, or litigation related to the deceased's death, or an intervening traumatic event or familial death (even if by natural causes), may retrigger traumatic reminders, excessive avoidance, anger, or other PTSD symptoms that had previously dissipated. Returning to trauma-focused interventions may be warranted in such situations.

In order to address trauma and grief issues sequentially, we present trauma-focused components and grief-focused components separately in this book. The grief-focused interventions we describe do not address how to treat children dealing with uncomplicated grief issues or children who have undergone traumatic experiences and separation from parents without death (e.g., placement in a foster home). Although some of the interventions in the grief-focused components may be applicable, loss associated with death is unique in that there is no hope of reunification in this life, as there may be when a child is placed in foster care or even in adoption. However, it should be noted that children in foster care have responded well to TF-CBT with modifications to address their special circumstances (e.g., including foster parents in treatment and/or addressing the stressors associated with foster placements).

SUMMARY

Although some children who experience traumatic events are resilient, many others develop trauma symptoms that can have a profound and long-lasting negative impact on their development, health, and safety. These trauma symptoms include affective, behavioral, and cognitive difficulties and may result in a diagnosis of PTSD, depressive or anxiety disorders, or "complex PTSD"; and even if the symptoms do not meet criteria for such disorders, they still have a significant negative impact on child and family functioning. Many of these children will also have psychobiological alterations in response to trauma. Children whose loved ones die in traumatic circumstances may develop CTG, a condition in which children are "stuck" on the traumatic circumstances of the death and cannot fully grieve the death of the loved one. The TF-CBT and grief-focused components described in this book help children with many of these types of difficulties. The next chapter focuses on assessing children who have experienced traumatic stress and/or traumatic grief reactions, and how to determine whether TF-CBT is the optimal treatment approach for a particular child.

CHAPTER 2

Assessment Strategies
for Traumatized Children

Although the TF-CBT model has broad applications, it is still important for clinicians to assess children and families for the presence of specific psychiatric disorders. Entities that fund treatment and certify treatment facilities require accurate diagnosis of existing psychopathology. Careful assessment is also essential for optimal treatment planning. Methods for conducting general child psychiatric evaluations are described in detail elsewhere (AACAP, 1997), and specific instruments and techniques for evaluating childhood PTSD are also available (AACAP, 1998). Here we discuss helpful strategies for assessing trauma exposure and trauma-related symptoms in children and adolescents.

EVALUATING TRAUMATIC EXPOSURE

Evaluating traumatic exposure is important in understanding the broader context of the child's life and is essential in assessing trauma symptoms that are typically referenced to the child's self-identified worst traumatic experience. Many clinicians include detailed inquiry about traumatic history in their routine assessment. Because childhood traumas are typically underreported and often co-occur (Saunders, 2003), routinely asking about traumatic history is recommended. Another option is to utilize a standardized format (either as an interview or a self- or parent-report instrument) that investigates a wide variety of childhood traumatic experiences. Examples include the UCLA PTSD Index for DSM-IV (Pynoos, Rodriguez, Steinberg, Stuber, & Fredrick, 1998) and the Traumatic Events Screening Inventory—Child Version (TESI-C; Ford et al., 1999). These instruments ask children to identify and rate the severity of each traumatic event they have experienced and to select the one that was most upsetting to them. This event is then used as the index trauma for rating trauma-related symptoms.

ASSESSING PTSD SYMPTOMS

Assessing PTSD symptoms may be accomplished in a variety of ways. Briefly, the diagnosis of PTSD requires that children have a specified number of symptoms in three distinct clusters:

- Reexperiencing: intrusive, upsetting thoughts or dreams about the traumatic event, physical or psychological distress upon exposure to reminders of the trauma; in young children, reenacting the traumatic event through play.
- Avoidance and emotional numbing: avoiding people, places, or situations that remind the child of the traumatic event; emotional detachment or flatness; sense of a foreshortened future.
- Hyperarousal and mood: increased startle reaction, hypervigilance, disturbed sleep, irritability, or angry outbursts.

Although the use of detailed semistructured interviews is the "gold standard" for evaluating the presence of these PTSD symptoms (AACAP, 1998), these are time- and labor-intensive, and few therapists in clinical settings have the resources to use these interviews on a regular basis. Several self-report instruments for assessing children's PTSD symptoms are available, which have acceptable reliability and validity for clinical use. These include the previously mentioned UCLA PTSD Index for DSM-IV (Pynoos, Rodriguez, et al., 1998), which is the most widely used child self-report measure for PTSD and has established scores for mild, moderate, severe, and very severe PTSD.

ASSESSING OTHER PSYCHIATRIC DISORDERS

Assessing for the possible presence of other psychiatric disorders is also essential. It is particularly important to evaluate whether children have active suicidal thoughts, intents, or plans or serious substance abuse, which might be transiently worsened during certain portions of the TF-CBT treatment model. Specifically, there are concerns that creating the trauma narrative may worsen suicidal ideation or substance abuse if it is already present in particularly fragile children. Thus it is critical to determine whether these conditions are present prior to starting the TF-CBT intervention, and if so, to use TF-CBT (or other) interventions aimed at enhancing affective regulation and stress reduction until the child has become more stabilized. Standard child psychiatric assessment procedures should be used to evaluate the presence of depression (including suicidality), substance use disorders, psychosis, and other psychiatric disorders (AACAP, 1997). It is particularly important to distinguish between true psychotic hallucinations and delusions and flashbacks or intrusive thoughts that may be symptoms of PTSD. Similarly, for children exhibiting severe behavioral difficulties (e.g., conduct disorder), it may be important to establish whether these conduct problems are linked, at least temporally, to the onset of the trauma. With many children, behavioral difficulties can be adequately addressed by working with parents on behavior management strategies and simultaneously teaching children emotional regulation strategies, as outlined in this model. However, other children, particularly those who have a long, pre-existing history of conduct problems or other self-destructive behaviors, may need a more extended period of treatment focused on emotional and behavioral stabilization before initiating TF-CBT. Clinicians will need to utilize their clinical judgment in determining whether treatment should initially focus on stabilizing the child's behavior prior to initiating any trauma-focused work. If the severe psychiatric conditions described above are either historical or current, these difficulties should be monitored and documented throughout the course of treatment. Prior to using trauma-focused interventions with such children, therapists should consider obtaining consultation with supervisors or others who are experienced in the use of the TF-CBT model.

It should be noted, however, that recent research suggests that children who have suffered multiple traumas and/or are experiencing significant depressive symptomatology may be less responsive to nondirective treatment approaches and may benefit more from the skill building, structure, and trauma-focused approach of TF-CBT (Deblinger et al., 2005).

As described in Chapter 1, traumatic experiences can affect children's functioning in a variety of domains. Thus, in addition to assessing for PTSD, during the initial evaluation sessions it is important to gather as much information as possible about the child's functioning across the domains described below. This information will contribute to the development of a case conceptualization that will then form the basis for designing an individually tailored TF-CBT treatment plan. TF-CBT components are designed to address many of these domains, which can be summarized by the acronym CRAFTS (for problem domains):

- Cognitive problems: Maladaptive patterns of thinking about self, others, and situations, including distortions or inaccurate thoughts (e.g., self-blame for traumatic events) and unhelpful thoughts (e.g., dwelling on the worst possibilities)
- Relationship problems: Difficulties getting along with peers, poor problem-solving or social skills, hypersensitivity in interpersonal interactions, maladaptive strategies for making friends, impaired interpersonal trust
- Affective problems: Sadness, anxiety, fear, anger, poor ability to tolerate or regulate negative affective states, inability to self-soothe
- Family problems: Parenting skill deficits, poor parent–child communication, disturbances in parent–child bonding, disruption in family function/relationships due to familial abuse or violence
- Traumatic behavior problems: Avoidance of trauma reminders; trauma-related, sexualized, aggressive, or oppositional behaviors; unsafe behaviors
- Somatic problems: Sleep difficulties, physiological hyperarousal and hypervigilance toward possible trauma cues, physical tension, somatic symptoms (headaches, stomachaches, etc.)

In addition to interviewing children and parents separately and relying on clinical observations to ascertain children's functioning in the above domains, there are some standardized measures that can provide objective assessments of children's adjustment levels in relation to the general population. Parents and/or teachers are typically the best resources for assessing a child's behavioral functioning. Two widely used child behavior measures include the Child Behavior Checklist (CBCL; Achenbach, 1991) and the Behavior Assessment System for Children (BASC; Reynolds & Kamphaus, 1992). These paper-and-pencil measures assess internalizing and externalizing symptomatology in children and adolescents and may be obtained in parent-report as well as teacher-report versions.

Although parents and teachers may provide the most accurate information regarding observable difficulties (e.g., acting-out behaviors, family and peer problems), children themselves are the best reporters of their own internal distress (Rev, Schrader, & Morris-Yates, 1992). Thus it is important to question children directly and/or utilize self-report standardized measures to assess for the possible presence of depression, anxiety, and/or other internal trauma symptoms in children and adolescents. Two general trauma symptom measures may be used: the Trauma Symptom Checklist for Children (Briere, 1995) and the Children's Impact of Events Scale (Wolfe, Gentile, Michienzi, Sas, & Wolfe, 1991). Self-report, normed measures utilized specifically to assess depression in children include the Children's Depression Inventory (Kovacs, 1985; ages 7–16), the Beck Youth Depression Inventory (Beck, Beck, & Jolly, 2001), and/or the Beck Depression Inventory–II (BDI-II; Beck, Steer, & Brown, 1996; ages 13 and older). Standardized self-report measures to assess anxiety in children and adolescents include the State–Trait Anxiety Inventory for Children (Spielberger, 1973), the Manifest Anxiety Scale for Children (MASC; March, Parker, Sullivan, Stallings, & Conners, 1997), and the Screen for Child Anxiety Related Emotional Disorders (SCARED) (Birmaher et al., 1997).

When possible, it is also helpful to get a good history of the child's coping style, adjustment, and functioning prior to the traumatic experience(s). Research suggests that children's psychosocial reactions to trauma may be moderated by their temperament, preexisting psychopathology, and their attributional or coping styles (Feiring, Taska, & Lewis, 2002; Spaccareli, 1994). Again, although this information can be obtained by interview, there are some measures that can assist particularly in terms of assessing trauma-related coping and attributional responses (Mannarino, Cohen, & Berman, 1994; Kolko, 1996).

Because a central aspect of TF-CBT treatment involves detailed discussions and/or writing about the identified traumatic event(s), it is helpful to assess the child's ability to offer a narrative about a positive life experience. Interestingly, Sternberg et al. (1997) found that when children were asked to give a detailed account of a neutral or positive event prior to being questioned about abuse allegations, their ability to offer details regarding the alleged abuse appeared to significantly increase. We have modified their approach to include giving children practice in sharing their feelings, thoughts, and even bodily sensations in relation to a positive or exciting experience (Deblinger, Behl, & Glickman, 2006). This assessment component provides children with an opportunity to practice skills that will become important as treatment proceeds. In addition, in the context of a treatment planning assessment, asking children to describe a favorite activity may help build rapport and provide a baseline expectation regarding their ability to articulate details and share associated thoughts, feelings, and sensations. Identifying children's skills in sharing a narrative about a favorite activity provides important information that may reflect developmental and cultural influences in terms of their comfort with, and language abilities for, articulating details and communicating with adults. A baseline narrative, for example, might reveal that the child has a very limited vocabulary for identifying feelings and is unable to offer more than three-word sentence descriptions about the favorite activity. This level of narrative would indicate the need for some skill building in relation to feeling expression; in regard to the level of detail expected during the trauma narrative, the therapist might need to adjust his/her expectations. In fact, the child should not be expected to do a highly detailed trauma narrative, but rather should be applauded for his/her efforts in developing a trauma narrative that is similar to the baseline narrative in terms of its depth and detail.

The child can be asked to share a baseline narrative during the evaluation and/or sometime prior to the initiation of the trauma-focused work by encouraging the sharing of such a narrative as follows:

THERAPIST: I'm really enjoying getting to know you, and I wondered if you would tell me about an activity you participated in recently that you really enjoyed. Can you tell me about a favorite activity or a party you went to recently that you enjoyed?

CHILD: Well, I could tell you about a birthday party I went to this weekend, but it wasn't that much fun.

THERAPIST: That's OK. I'd like to hear about it anyway.

CHILD: OK.

THERAPIST: I didn't go to that birthday party, so could you tell me all about it? Tell me everything that happened from the time you arrived to the time the birthday cake was brought out. And maybe you could tell me how you were feeling and what you were saying to yourself during the party?

As much as possible, allow the child to provide a spontaneous narrative. However, when there are very long pauses or the child gets significantly off task, you may jump in with one of the questions or statements below.

1. Ask broad, open-ended questions:
   "What were you thinking?"
   "What were you saying to yourself?"
   "How were you feeling?"
   "What happened next?"

2. Make clarifying and reflective statements:
   "Tell me more about it. . . . "
   "I wasn't there, so tell me. . . . "
   "I want to know all about. . . . "
   "Repeat the part about. . . . "
   Repeat this exercise, this time applying it to a traumatic experience.

THERAPIST: Can you tell me why your mom brought you to see me?

CHILD: I think she wants me to talk to you about what happened when the police took my dad away.

THERAPIST: I'd like you to tell me more about that. You did such a good job telling me all about what happened at the birthday party. Now I'd like you tell me about everything that happened on the day the police came to your house. Would you like to tell me about what was happening before the police came or what happened after the police came to your house?

CHILD: I'll tell you what happened after the police came 'cause I don't think you want to hear the scary stuff that happened before they came.

THERAPIST: I'd like to hear about the scary stuff too, but today I'd like you to tell me everything that happened from the time the police arrived at your house until they left with your dad. And please tell me what you were feeling and what you were saying to yourself while all this was happening.

CHILD: OK. I'll try.

This initial trauma narrative may also be considered a baseline because it may provide you with some information about how avoidant the child is prior to working with him/her on any emotional regulation or stress management skills. It is important during this initial discussion of the trauma to accept whatever the child offers by asking the types of open-ended questions suggested above. In this early stage it is not necessary to push the child for further details. Rather, it is more important to focus on building rapport and on praising the child for sharing whatever he/she managed to reveal.

Research strongly suggests that parents' levels of distress can significantly influence children's reactions to trauma as well as their responsiveness to treatment (Cohen & Mannarino, 1996b, 2000; Deblinger, Lippmann, & Steer, 1996; Spaccareli, 1994). Thus, although parents participate in TF-CBT treatment on behalf of their children and are not considered direct recipients of treatment for personal difficulties (e.g., unrelated work or marital distress), it is critical to assess their adjustment and ability to serve as effective role models and support resources for their child(ren) during and after the treatment process. It is therefore important to obtain historical information about parents' trauma exposure and their own psychosocial responses. Interviewing the parent about the circumstances and impact of the trauma(s) offers information about the parent's coping ability and may help to identify the aspects of the trauma that the child and/or parent may find most difficult to discuss. This information may be particularly useful when initiating the trauma-focused work. There are also several measures that are useful in assessing parents' trauma-specific reactions: the Impact of Events Scale (Joseph, Williams, Yule, & Walker, 1992), the Parental Emotional Reaction Questionnaire (Mannarino & Cohen, 1996), and the UCLA PTSD Index for DSM-IV (Pynoos, Rodriguez, et al., 1998) cited above. In addition, there are numerous standardized measures available to assess parents' levels of general symptomatology (BDI-II; Beck et al., 1996; Symptom Checklist–90 [SCL-90]; Derogatis, Lipman, & Covi, 1973).

As indicated above with regard to the children, it is also critical to screen for the presence of serious psychiatric conditions in the parent(s). In some instances, the treatment planning assessment may reveal the parents' limited capacity to participate due to active substance abuse difficulties, severe mental health difficulties (e.g., active psychosis or suicidality), and/or behaviors (i.e., physically abusive) that put children at risk. Prior to initiating TF-CBT, these issues should be addressed with effective case management, clinical referrals, and/or reports to the appropriate agency (e.g., child protection) when required by state law. Although participation by a supportive adult is optimal for the child, research does indicate that children can benefit from TF-CBT, particularly in terms of overcoming PTSD, even if no adult actively participates on their behalf (Deblinger et al., 1996). In addition, with the consent of the legal guardian, the child may benefit from the participation of another supportive adult such as a grandparent, stepparent, aunt, foster parent, etc.

ASSESSMENT OF CHILDHOOD TRAUMATIC GRIEF

In the clinical assessment of CTG, it is important to obtain information directly from the child as well as from the parents or other primary caretaker. Several protocols for evaluating grieving children (Webb, 2002; Fox, 1985) provide guidance for obtaining information about the nature of the death, mourning rituals, etc. The current conceptualization of CTG requires (1) that the loved one died under circumstances that the child perceived to be traumatic (horrifying, shocking, terrifying); (2) the presence of significant PTSD symptoms, including that trauma, loss, and change reminders segue into thoughts about the traumatic cause of the death; and (3) that these PTSD symptoms impinge on the child's ability to complete the tasks of reconciliation. The following sections focus on gathering information about these areas.

Traumatic Nature of the Death

In most cases of CTG, the loved one died in an objectively traumatic manner, that is, one that was sudden, violent, and gory (e.g., gunshot, hanging, motor vehicle accident, explosion, fire). However, in some instances, the loved one died of natural causes, but the death was subjectively traumatic to the child because it was totally unexpected (e.g., heart attack or stroke), was accompanied by characteristics that caused the child to feel shock and helplessness (e.g., the person collapsed, bled profusely, vomited, turned blue), or was perceived by the child to be unbearably agonizing to the deceased (e.g., gasping for breath, screaming in pain, begging for help).

As part of the National Child Traumatic Stress Network's Child Traumatic Grief Work Group, the Prevalence and Correlates Subcommittee developed two interviews that can be used to gather information about the child's and surviving parent's experience of the loved one's death. These interviews—characteristics, attributions, and responses after exposure to death (CARED–Child and Parent Versions; Brown, Cohen, Amaya-Jackson, Handel, & Layne, 2003)—are the first instruments of this type that have been developed in the CTG field.

The Presence of PTSD Symptoms with Relation to the Death

We described how to evaluate children's PTSD symptoms earlier in this chapter. Briefly, it is essential to inquire about these symptoms specifically in relation to the loved one's death, in a manner that is developmentally appropriate, and to obtain this information from both the child and parent because some symptoms are more easily observed and reported by parents (e.g., irritability, traumatic play) and others require self-report by the child (e.g., intrusive thoughts, avoidance, sense of a foreshortened future).

Impingement of PTSD Symptoms on Grieving

The critical factor here is whether thoughts or reminders of the deceased segue into trauma reminders in such a manner that the child gets stuck in remembering the horrifying manner in which the person died and therefore avoids thinking about the deceased in positive ways. It may be helpful to use specific examples in asking children about this area (e.g., "When you see pictures of your sister, are you able to remember mostly happy times, or do you keep thinking about what she looked like at the moment she was shot?" or "Do you find that sometimes you try not to think about your father at all? Is that because every time you think of him, you start remembering the fire in which he died?"). It is also helpful to inquire about how often the child thinks about the deceased (if rarely, is this an effort to avoid trauma reminders?; if frequently, what proportion of the time do these thoughts segue into traumatic memories, and what is the child's reaction to these traumatic memories?), and what, if anything, interrupts this process (is it sadness associated with uncomplicated bereavement, or terrifying images about the traumatic cause of death and/or the deceased's suffering?). Does the child avoid previously enjoyed activities because doing them reminds him/her of the deceased? Does the child avoid people who remind him/her of the deceased? It is also usually helpful to ask the parent or other primary caretaker these questions as well, because highly avoidant children may respond negatively to such questions even if these symptoms are present.

There is currently only one empirically validated instrument for measuring CTG. This instrument, the Expanded Grief Inventory (EGI; Layne, Savjak, Saltzman, & Pynoos, 2001), has 28 items that cover both uncomplicated bereavement and CTG. Factor analysis of this instrument performed by the authors identified four distinct factors: Positive Connection (reflective of the child's ability to have positive reminiscences of the deceased), Existentially Complicated Grief (indicative of emptiness resulting from the death), Traumatic Intrusion and Avoidance (referring to the intrusion of trauma symptoms on the child's ability to reminisce or have positive feelings about the deceased), and a fourth unnamed factor encompassing items that did not correlate highly with the other three (Layne, Savjak, et al., 2001). These factor analyses were conducted from data collected on Bosnian adolescents exposed to war-related trauma and loss, as well as Los Angeles youth exposed to community violence. Subsequent factor analyses by Brown and Goodman (2005), conducted with children who lost firefighter parents following 9/11, revealed two main factors rather than four. These factors roughly corresponded to uncomplicated bereavement and CTG symptoms. Further testing and development of the EGI, and possibly other instruments measuring CTG in younger children, are needed to improve our ability to quantify symptoms of this condition.

Finally, researchers have developed an instrument to evaluate complicated grief in adults, which can be used to assess the presence of these symptoms in parents who have lost their spouses, partners, or children under traumatic circumstances. This instrument is called the Inventory of Complicated Grief (ICG; Prigerson et al., 1995) and can be used to evaluate these symptoms in parents of children with CTG.

PROVIDING FEEDBACK TO THE FAMILY ABOUT THE ASSESSMENT

Prior to initiating treatment, it is important to present the assessment findings and treatment conceptualization to parents as well as to children, when appropriate. Summarizing the assessment findings can be very reassuring to parents, who may be unsure as to whether you fully appreciate the impact of the trauma on their lives, individually and as a family. Specific diagnoses may be presented, but parents may find straightforward explanations of diagnoses and standardized scores more meaningful and less frightening and stigmatizing. It is also critically important to incorporate the child's identified strengths into the presentation of the assessment findings. In fact, the therapist should present the treatment plan in terms of how it will specifically address the difficulties identified in the assessment and how it will capitalize on the child's and parents' strengths. It is particularly helpful at this stage to emphasize the powerful influence parental support can have on a child's trauma recovery, thereby highlighting the important role parents play in the treatment process. By providing a treatment overview and explaining the structure of treatment in terms of the individual sessions for children and parents, followed by conjoint parent–child sessions, you can further emphasize the expectation that, as parents, they will be the most valuable therapeutic resources for their children during conjoint sessions and, more importantly, when formal therapy sessions end. Whenever possible, parents are given general expectations in terms of the number of sessions (e.g., 12–18 sessions) and/or the appropriate time frame for the completion of treatment. This information can be reassuring to parents and children and may enhance their likelihood to make a commitment to a full course of treatment.

In order to encourage parents to talk openly and to freely ask questions, children should not be present while the therapist is presenting the assessment findings to the parents. However, depending on the child's age, it may be helpful for the therapist to present the findings to the child in terms of what was learned from the assessment about his/her difficulties as well as strengths. Then, in simple and concrete terms, the therapist can present a brief description of the treatment plan specifically in terms of how it will help the child overcome some of the difficulties identified. Again, the therapist should avoid overwhelming the child with too much information, but rather should focus on inspiring confidence that therapy will build on his/her family's strengths and help all members cope effectively with the trauma experienced.

Finally, it should be noted that ongoing informal assessment should continue throughout treatment to guide the process, particularly in terms of identifying coping skills deficits and cognitive distortions, planning the trauma-focused work, and effectively timing conjoint and family sessions. A posttreatment assessment, ideally incorporating the standardized measures administered at pretreatment, should be conducted shortly before the planned termination. Although TF-CBT has demonstrated excellent success in helping children and parents regain their equilibrium and overcome PTSD, this does not mean 100% removal of symptoms occurs every time. Clinicians should not postpone termination because a complete resolution of trauma-related symptoms has not been achieved. In fact, recent research suggests that children and parents often demonstrate improvement beyond the termination of treatment as they continue to utilize their skills and gain healthier perspectives on their survival of the traumatic experience(s) (Deblinger et al., 2005). Moreover, it is likely that some impact of the trauma will always be felt, and this experience is not necessarily unhealthy. In sum, the posttreatment assessment should be utilized to document and celebrate treatment progress while also verifying the general appropriateness of the discharge plan, with the proviso that children and parents may return for therapy if the need arises.

CHAPTER 3

The TF-CBT Model
How It Works

The rest of this book describes TF-CBT, an empirically supported treatment model designed to assist children, adolescents, and their parents in the aftermath of traumatic experiences. TF-CBT is a components-based hybrid approach that integrates trauma-sensitive interventions, cognitive-behavioral principles, as well as aspects of attachment, developmental neurobiology, family, empowerment, and humanistic theoretical models in order to optimally address the needs of traumatized children and families.

TF-CBT components particularly address symptoms of PTSD, depression, and anxiety, as well as features associated with these conditions. Although TF-CBT components can address and successfully resolve certain behavioral problems, it may not be ideally suited for children whose *primary* difficulties reflect severe preexisting behavioral difficulties.

Core values of the TF-CBT model can be summarized by the acronym CRAFTS (for core values):

- Components based
- Respectful of cultural values
- Adaptable and flexible
- Family focused
- Therapeutic relationship is central
- Self-efficacy is emphasized

Components-based treatment emphasizes a set of central skills that progressively build on previously consolidated skills. Rather than describe a rigid session-by-session treatment approach, TF-CBT describes interrelated components, each of which should be provided in a manner, intensity, and duration that best matches the needs of the individual child and family.

Respect for individual, family, religious, community, and cultural values is essential for any psychosocial intervention to work effectively. TF-CBT therapists work together with the child and parent to decide the best way to implement the core components for their family, with an awareness that this treatment must occur in harmony with the family's larger community and cultural context.

Adaptability is crucial to the success of the TF-CBT model. Therapists must be creative and flexible in implementing the core components of this treatment. The individual therapist's clinical judgment and creativity are highly valued and respected in this approach and ultimately determines how the TF-CBT components are used to help each child and family.

Family involvement is one of the most important features of the TF-CBT model. Parents are integrally included in the child's treatment, and a primary focus of treatment is improving parent–child interactions, communication, and closeness. Siblings may also be included in treatment when clinically appropriate.

Therapeutic relationships are central to the TF-CBT approach. We believe that developing and maintaining trusting, accepting, empathic therapeutic relationships with their therapist is essential to restoring trust, optimism and self-esteem in traumatized children and their parents.

Self-efficacy, including self-regulation of affect, behavior, and cognitions, is a long-term goal of the TF-CBT approach. TF-CBT aims to provide life skills and enhance individual strengths so that children, parents, and families continue to thrive long after therapy has ended.

DEVELOPMENT OF THE TF-CBT MODEL

The treatment model described here reflects our ongoing commitment to the development and evaluation of interventions designed to optimally address the mental health needs of children and parents suffering from traumatic stress and/or grief. From early on, beginning almost two decades ago, our clinical work and research investigations have been focused on understanding the difficulties faced by traumatized children (Cohen & Mannarino, 1998a, 1998b; Deblinger, McLeer, Atkins, Ralph, & Foa, 1989) and designing interventions that would ameliorate the problems identified (Deblinger, McLeer, & Henry, 1990; Cohen & Mannarino, 1993). We have conducted several pre–post investigations (Deblinger et al., 1990; Stauffer & Deblinger, 1996; Cohen, Mannarino, & Staron, 2005) and five randomized controlled trials demonstrating the efficacy of the TF-CBT model (Cohen & Mannarino, 1996a, 1998a; Cohen, Deblinger, et al., 2004; Deblinger et al., 1996; Deblinger, Stauffer, & Steer, 2001). In addition, the efficacy of TF-CBT and similar CBT treatment models for children who have suffered traumatic stress has been replicated by other researchers (King et al., 2000; March, Amaya-Jackson, Murray, & Schulte, 1998). Although there are many approaches to treatment that are likely to be valuable for children who have suffered trauma, recent reviews of the child sexual abuse treatment outcome literature have documented that TF-CBT appears to have the most rigorous empirical support for its effectiveness in treating PTSD and related difficulties in this population of children (AACAP, 1998; Putnam, 2003; Saunders, Berliner, & Hanson, 2004; modelprograms. samhsa.gov). Because of its proven efficacy in treating symptoms and difficulties frequently associated with traumatic stress and grief, TF-CBT for children and parents is being applied and empirically evaluated with children who have suffered a wide array of traumatic experiences (e.g., traumatic grief, exposure to domestic or community violence).

This book is the culmination of a longstanding collaboration of clinical researchers in Pittsburgh (Cohen and Mannarino) and New Jersey (Deblinger) who had previously independently developed and tested trauma-focused treatment manuals for sexually abused preschoolers and school-age children/adolescents (Deblinger & Heflin, 1996; Cohen & Mannarino, 1992, 1994). Although these treatment manuals overlapped in many ways, they placed somewhat different emphases on different components.

Deblinger's previously published treatment manual, identified as a cognitive-behavioral model, pioneered the use of gradual exposure techniques with traumatized children (Deblinger & Heflin, 1996). These techniques included *in vivo* exposure to feared trauma reminders as well as encouraging children to describe and/or write about the details of their traumatic experiences and the associated thoughts, feelings, and sensations. Deblinger also emphasized the potential therapeutic role parents could play by encouraging their participation in conjoint sessions with their children. Although Cohen and Mannarino's earlier treatment manuals were grounded in cognitive-behavioral principles, they attempted to integrate aspects of other theoretical frameworks as well. Their component-based manuals included an emphasis on (1) the meaning of the abuse in the context of the child's relationships to the perpetrator and nonoffender parent (attachment and family impact), (2) the child's degree of interpersonal trust and self-efficacy (empowerment), and (3) how the child's abuse experience, and in many cases the mother's previous abuse, were reflected in the child's and parents' relationships with others. Additionally, Cohen and Mannarino have directed a program for children who have experienced many types of trauma besides, or in addition to, sexual abuse, including traumatic grief. They and their colleagues have developed a treatment manual for childhood traumatic grief (Cohen, Greenberg, et al., 2001) based on several years' experience of treating children who have experienced the traumatic death of a parent or sibling.

With the development, funding, and implementation of a collaborative multisite study in 1997, we merged our similar approaches into an integrated treatment model, which has been empirically evaluated most rigorously with sexually abused, multiply traumatized, and traumatically bereaved children, but has also been extensively used clinically at our centers with children who have experienced other types of traumatic life events and is now being empirically tested specifically for children who have experienced domestic violence. Through Cohen and Mannarino's early work in the National Child Traumatic Stress Network (NCTSN), we have extensively modified this book to include many suggestions made by community therapists affiliated with the NCTSN and with the Child and Adolescent Treatment and Services (CATS) Consortium in New York City, which was started after the terrorist attacks on September 11, 2001.

INDIVIDUAL CHILD AND CONJOINT PARENT TREATMENT MODEL

TF-CBT incorporates individual child and parent sessions as well as conjoint sessions. There is evidence from controlled (Stein et al., 2003; Kataoka et al., 2003; Chemtob, Nakashima, & Hamada, 2002), quasi-controlled (Goenjian et al., 1997), and open studies (i.e., studies without a control or comparison group; March et al., 1998; Layne, Pynoos, et al., 2001) that group therapy is effective in resolving PTSD and other trauma symptoms in children. Moreover, there are some situations in which group therapy is the *only* practical possibility (e.g., in war-torn countries where there are many children affected and few therapists available). However, it is more typical in community practices to receive individual referrals of traumatized children one at a time. Therapists who have tried to organize group interventions in these settings are familiar with the difficulties faced in finding a sufficient number of children of similar developmental levels, all of whom experienced the same type of traumatic stressor, to come to treatment at the same time on the same day. In addition, there are logistical problems, such as the kids who miss sessions and end up out of synchrony with the rest of the group. Individual therapy eliminates these complexities and allows the therapist to tailor treatment to each individual child and family's needs. Additionally, although it appears that there are specific benefits to group therapy (e.g., diminishing stigma by participating in therapy with peers who have had similar traumatic experiences; increasing the potential for developing more appropriate cognitions by hearing other children's perspectives on their traumatic experience), there are also potential pitfalls that are avoided by providing treatment individually (e.g., children being retraumatized by hearing detailed descriptions of events they themselves did not experience; the concern about "tainting" children's legal testimony through hearing other children's accounts of traumatic events). We believe it is important to provide an individual treatment approach for those clinicians who choose to provide, and families who prefer to receive, this form of intervention. However, it should be noted that modified versions of TF-CBT have been implemented in the group therapy format as well (Stauffer & Deblinger, 1996; Deblinger et al., 2001).

Parents are often traumatized themselves, either directly or vicariously, by the child's traumatic experience. For example, nonoffending parents of children exposed to domestic violence are themselves direct victims of that violence; parents of children traumatized by community disasters such as floods, hurricanes, or terrorism have also experienced these events and may have their own trauma symptoms. Including parents in therapy provides such parents with trauma-focused components that may help them cope better as well as allowing them to optimally encourage their children in practicing these skills. In fact, the findings of our multisite investigation documented that TF-CBT was effective in helping nonoffending parents overcome depressive symptoms as well as abuse-specific distress (Cohen, Deblinger, et al., 2004).

Still, it should be emphasized that this TF-CBT model is *child focused*. Although some of the parent's personal symptoms and difficulties may be addressed in this process, those who are experiencing severe PTSD or other significant psychiatric symptoms may need referral to individual treatment (psychotherapy and possibly pharmacotherapy) for adequate resolution. Referral is especially important if the parent's symptoms are significantly impairing his/her emotional availability or judgment to the point that the therapist believes it is interfering with adequate parenting practices. The therapist should address these concerns directly with the parent in a supportive and nonjudgmental manner.

The parent interventions are presented in this book in the same order as the child interventions. The therapist should be flexible in adjusting this sequence in order to parallel each child's treatment as well as to address parental issues that arise during the course of therapy. This parallel format informs the parent of the content covered in each child session, thereby optimally preparing the parent to reinforce this material with the child between sessions. It is helpful to start each parent session by asking about any successes with between-session therapy assignments in order to consistently emphasize the importance of the parent's efforts at home. However, there may be situations in which the parent needs a different (rather than parallel) component from the child, and the TF-CBT model allows for this flexibility.

Although several group treatment approaches (particularly those carried out in school settings) have not included a parental treatment component (e.g., Layne, Pynoos, et al., 2001; March et al., 1998; Stein et al., 2003; Goenjian et al., 1997), we believe that including parents in treatment is optimally helpful for most traumatized children. Just as psychological difficulties can be greatly influenced by environmental factors, recovery from trauma-related problems can be facilitated or impeded by children's environments. The most immediate and influential environment for most children is that of their families. Parents can have an important impact on whether, to what degree, and how quickly children recover from trauma-related problems. They can also influence whether children's improvements are temporary (i.e., only for the time that the child is in treatment) or whether these gains are sustained long after the end of treatment. We view parents as an important source of support and reinforcement for children's progress both during treatment and subsequently. Including parents in treatment is an optimal means by which to attain TF-CBT goals of enhancing parenting efficacy, parent–child communication, and familial attachments. Specifically, participation by both parties in this relationship (e.g., child and parent) has the best chance of effecting lasting positive changes in that relationship. Thus, for many reasons, we believe that parent inclusion is a critical component for children's recovery from trauma symptoms.

There is also scientific evidence that actively including parents in TF-CBT is helpful. One study directly examined the impact of including a parent component (Deblinger et al., 1996) by randomly assigning children who had suffered sexual abuse to one of four treatment conditions: TF-CBT for the child only, TF-CBT for the parent only, TF-CBT for both child and parent, and referral to treatment as usual in the community. This study demonstrated that providing treatment to the parent resulted in significantly greater improvement in the child's depressive and externalizing behavioral symptoms, *even when the child was not seen individually in treatment.* Additionally, parents assigned to therapy conditions that required their active participation in treatment demonstrated significantly greater improvement in their parenting practices.

Another study reported that including a family treatment component resulted in lower levels of abuse-related fears in children 3 months after treatment had ended (King et al., 2000). Two other studies indirectly evaluated the benefit of including parents in treatment. Cohen and Mannarino (1996b) found that for young (3- to 7-year-old) sexually abused children, the nonoffending parent's emotional distress related to the child's abuse was a strong predictor of treatment response immediately after treatment. Twelve months after treatment had ended, parental support of the child significantly predicted the child's degree of symptomatology as well (Cohen & Mannarino, 1998b). In a similar study of older children (8- to 14-year-olds), we found that parental support was also a strong predictor of treatment response (Cohen & Mannarino, 2000). Our recent studies of multiply traumatized children (Cohen, Deblinger, et al., 2004) and traumatically bereaved children (Cohen, Mannarino, & Knudsen, 2004) demonstrated that TF-CBT interventions not only resulted in improvement in children's symptoms but also in participating parents' personal PTSD and depressive symptoms, even though the focus of parental treatment in both of these studies was on the child's problems rather than on the parents' personal symptomatology. There is growing evidence from studies of children exposed to other types of trauma that less parental distress and more familial support mitigate the negative impact of trauma on children (Laor et al., 2001; Kliewer et al., 2001). Thus interventions that help the parent resolve emotional distress about the child's trauma and optimize the parent's ability to be supportive of the child are likely to improve the child's outcome beyond whatever interventions are provided directly to the child.

Some therapists have raised concerns about confidentiality (i.e., whether it is ethical to share information about the child's or adolescent's treatment with parents). As a general rule, this treatment model is designed to encourage healthy open communication within families. However, we recognize the importance of obtaining consent from older children and adolescents before sharing such information. Nonetheless, we have almost never had the experience of a patient absolutely refusing to allow us to share any information with a parent. We have had adolescents ask that certain information be kept private, and unless safety issues were present, we have respected this request. We have found it helpful to explore with children the underlying concerns they have had about sharing trauma-related information with their parents; almost always these concerns were *not* related to confidentiality but were rather concerns about causing the parent greater emotional distress or fear that the parent would blame or punish the child for something the child had done or not done related to the traumatic event. Such exploration has allowed us to identify children's cognitive distortions (e.g., the belief that the parent blamed the child for being traumatized) and to help us and the parents address the source of the child's distress.

For example, in a sexual abuse case, the perpetrator gave the child money and gifts after abusive episodes. This child was afraid to share this information with his mother for fear she would blame him for the abuse or accuse him of colluding with the abuser. The therapist told the child that she did not believe his mother would feel this way if the mother understood the situation, and asked the child if she could explore this with the mother. This child was apprehensive about the mother finding out, but he was also relieved that the therapist did not think the mother would blame him, and that the therapist would talk to the mother about it instead of the child having to do so himself. Although the mother was initially upset to learn that her child had accepted gifts from the perpetrator, she was able to cognitively process her reaction with the therapist and could be very supportive of the child when they met together in conjoint sessions. Thus including parents in treatment is often of critical importance in resolving the child's trauma related problems.

On the other hand, it is important to recognize developmental differences between adolescents and younger children, and to encourage age-appropriate independence and separation/individuation from parental authority while also encouraging and enhancing appropriate parent–adolescent communication and parental support of the traumatized adolescent. Certain issues may be appropriately kept private during therapy with adolescents, whereas others may be appropriate to share. For example, teens may understandably not want to share every detail of their dating experiences with parents, and the therapist should help parents to recognize that it is age-appropriate for adolescents to desire and expect some privacy in this regard, as long as inappropriate or abusive behaviors are not occurring. Parental respect for age-appropriate boundaries and privacy for adolescents may enhance the quality and depth of trust between parent and adolescent as their relationship is successfully nurtured during the course of therapy.

As noted earlier, except for days when conjoint child–parent sessions are conducted (or when behavioral problems dictate joint meetings to develop joint strategies to address these), parents and children typically meet individually with the therapist each week. We have included a parent intervention section in each of the TF-CBT components. Generally, parents and children utilize parallel components in any given treatment session. However, as noted, there may be situations in which therapists provide one component to the child and a different component to the parent.

There may be situations in which a parent cannot or will not agree to be involved in treatment (e.g., if a child is in a group home, if foster parents refuse to participate, if the child's single parent has died and the child has been placed in a temporary shelter setting, if the child is a "street person"). Although inclusion of a parent or caretaker is optimal, we have provided TF-CBT to children only, as in the Deblinger et al. (1996) study, which demonstrated significant improvement in PTSD symptoms. Thus, while we strongly advocate that parents or other caretaking adults participate in this treatment, we also acknowledge that children may benefit even in the absence of parental involvement.

THE IMPORTANCE OF CULTURE IN THE TF-CBT MODEL

Although studies have shown that PTSD occurs across diverse cultures, cultural factors can affect how this disorder is manifested (Ahmad & Mohamad, 1996; DiNicola, 1996; Jenkins & Bell, 1994). For example, some Latino children may manifest PTSD symptoms as *susto* ("fright" or "soul loss"), an illness that is attributed to a frightening event that causes the soul to leave the body, resulting in somatic symptoms, sleep and appetite disturbances, sadness, poor self-esteem, and impaired functioning (APA, 2000). Latino families may attribute different meanings to dreams of deceased loved ones than other cultures, and traumatically bereaved Latino children may thus react differently to such dreams than other traumatically bereaved children. Native Americans may develop *ghost sickness*, a preoccupation with death and a deceased person resulting in bad dreams, feelings of danger, fear, hopelessness, and symptoms of panic (APA, 2000).

Additionally, different cultural and religious groups have their own traditions and rituals for coping with trauma and stress. Given the children's home base and the likely influence both family and community have on the way they manifest distress and access support, it is essential that therapists treating traumatized children understand the broader context of their world (Cohen, Deblinger, Mannarino, & De Arellano, 2001). The therapist should discuss these issues directly with the parent and, in some cases, with the child as well. This knowledge helps the therapist apply the TF-CBT interventions in a manner that respects and benefits from the child's culture and religion. Therapists obviously cannot change their own culture, nor will they belong to the same cultural milieu of all the children whom they treat, but they can still function as a source of support and healing to each child. Alicia Lieberman (personal communication, December 2003) refers to the "symphony of support" that ideally surrounds traumatized children: The therapist is only one component in this symphony, with the family and community providing the cultural context in which the child can heal and grow. It is also important for therapists to recognize and respect the universality of traumatic reactions as well as the pain that trauma causes to children and the families who care for them.

OPTIMIZING ADAPTIVE FUNCTIONING: THE IMPORTANCE OF ADJUNCTIVE SERVICES

In order to optimize adaptive functioning (i.e., the ability to function optimally in one's family, with friends and peers at school, in a state of physical and emotional health), it is important to prevent or minimize secondary adversities. In the context of a traumatic event, these adversities may include any psychological, financial, legal, medical, or other situation that arises either as a result of the traumatic event itself or secondary to the child's or parent's trauma-related reactions.

Few people are informed about or prepared for the complexities of legal and administrative actions that need to be completed following many traumatic events. In the case of sexual abuse, multiple agencies are typically involved in investigative, child protective, and law enforcement procedures following the child's disclosure of abuse. Domestic violence cases may require involvement with magistrates, child protection services, police, victim advocacy organizations, and other programs in order to obtain and enforce protective orders. In a fire or explosion, the family may have lost their home and crucial financial or legal documents (e.g., financial records, checkbooks, credit cards). Motor vehicle accidents may result in loss of transportation as well as criminal and civil legal proceedings. The unanticipated traumatic death of the family's wage earner or some disaster situations may impinge on a family's ability to access essentials such as food, electricity, mortgage payments, etc. Any of these traumatic events may also involve serious physical injuries, hospitalizations, and ongoing medical expenses.

These secondary adversities are further complicated in cases of traumatic death when the remains are not located or identified for a prolonged period of time, as in the case of the 2001 terrorist attacks on the United States and the 2004 tsunami in southeast Asia, or when release of victims' names is delayed, as was the case in the 1994 crash of USAir Flight 427 in Pittsburgh (Stubenbort, Donnelly, & Cohen, 2001). Locating financial records, gaining access to the deceased's financial assets, settling the deceased's estate, accessing insurance benefits, etc., are all potentially difficult tasks under the best of circumstances; CTG may impair the surviving parent's ability to complete these tasks in a timely manner, which may negatively affect the family's financial situation.

Finally, it is important to recognize the special needs of children who have lost both parents or a single parent who was their sole caretaker. These children have experienced not only trauma and loss of parent(s), but also are likely to be displaced from their home, school, peers, and/or community as a result of going to live with relatives or foster parents. Because these children are deprived of the parental support and stability that normally assists children in adapting to such large-scale changes, they have even greater challenges to overcome. Assuring placement with a competent caretaker—preferably with a relative or family friend with whom the child is comfortable and who knew the deceased parent(s)—should be the first priority. The new caretaker also faces significant challenges, both practical (financial, arranging legal custody, dealing with new schools, pediatricians, adjusting family routines to accommodate a child raised with different routines) and emotional (adjusting to being the caretaker for a traumatized and bereaved child). Therapists may assist the new family by helping to establish optimal communication between the child and new caretaker (e.g., facilitating flexibility in the child and caretaker[s] in adjusting to each others' rules, expectations). Although these issues are discussed in the section on parenting skills, they may need to be addressed throughout the course of treatment.

It is imperative that parents be provided with the information and resources to address these needs. In some cases the therapist may be the most readily available source of such information. For this reason, therapists treating traumatized children should familiarize themselves with resources such as state-run Victims Compensation services, the American Red Cross (which provides emergency food, shelter, and clothing for survivors of fires or other disaster situations), free or reduced-fee legal aid services, Aid for Dependent Children (food stamps, etc.), and other social service agencies that address these areas. In some cases the therapist will need to advocate for the child in nontherapeutic settings (e.g., assisting school personnel in recognizing traumatic behaviors in the child that may be impairing his/her ability to function in school). These interventions are not formally included in the TF-CBT treatment components, but they may be as important to the child's recovery as any other interventions the therapist provides.

Children with preexisting psychiatric or medical conditions may experience exacerbations of these difficulties following exposure to a traumatic event. Children with preexisting anxiety disorders, in particular, are more vulnerable to developing PTSD following traumatic exposure (LaGreca, Silverman, & Wasserstein, 1998). In order to prevent secondary adversities related to these conditions (e.g., school phobia, school failure, violent or aggressive behaviors), therapists should have experience in diagnosing the full spectrum of child psychiatric disorders and providing appropriate treatments and/or referral resources.

GENERAL CONSIDERATIONS IN USING THIS BOOK

In the rest of this book we describe each of the TF-CBT and grief-focused components separately. Certain of these components may be more relevant or helpful than others to an individual child or family. Although we present the TF-CBT as distinct components for teaching purposes, in practice the components build on and interface with each other. Clinical judgment is important in deciding which component to introduce or focus on at which times in the therapeutic process, and how long to spend on a specific component before progressing to another component. Once a particular component has been introduced in therapy, it may be revisited at later points in the treatment; these skills have broad applicability for a wide range of situations children and families may encounter.

We introduce the TF-CBT components in an order that progressively builds on skills and concepts learned earlier in the book. For example, we introduce relaxation and other affective modulation skills prior to the skill of creating the child's trauma narrative because the former skills help children feel more confident that they can tolerate telling their trauma story. However, it should be noted that some children do not necessarily require relaxation training prior to engaging in trauma-focused work, because they may be fairly comfortable talking about the trauma, but they may need to develop emotional and cognitive expressive skills in order to effectively share their thoughts and feelings. Similarly, the trauma narrative is typically created before the traumatic experience is cognitively processed because the child's cognitive distortions are often first expressed during the narrative process. Indeed, it is preferable to avoid focusing on correcting these distortions until a fair amount of the narrative has been written, so that children do not start censoring their narrative, but rather share what they were actually feeling and thinking at the time of the trauma. Clinical judgment and the child's individual situation, however, may dictate that an alternative order be used in introducing the TF-CBT components. This flexibility in sequencing is consistent with the TF-CBT model as long as all appropriate TF-CBT components are utilized at some point in the therapy process.

It is also important to recognize that in many clinical situations, aspects of several components can be blended together in a single session to provide an optimal intervention. For example, children having problems with peer or sibling relationships may need to utilize cognitive processing, affective modulation, relaxation, and behavioral skills in order to improve these relationships; effective parenting strategies will also likely contribute to positive changes in this regard. How and when to blend the various TF-CBT components depends on the therapist's skill and clinical judgment.

The TF-CBT components themselves also overlap to some degree and, in many cases, we made arbitrary decisions regarding which intervention was included in which component in the book. For example, we included relaxation as a separate component, in part, to provide specific interventions that target somatic symptoms. However, relaxation is also an important affective modulation skill, so this separation is somewhat artificial. Similarly, cognitive strategies are important tools for affective self-soothing but are included as a separate component. In fact, this component also becomes critical in the latter stages of the trauma narrative component, when children are encouraged to examine, process, and correct cognitive distortions and developing beliefs.

Since TF-CBT is a skills- and strengths-based model, its components typically need to be practiced by the child and parent in order to be optimally effective. We therefore provide the acronym *PRACTICE* to remind the child and family (and therapist) of the core TF-CBT components and the value of practicing them for the duration of treatment and beyond. In fact, some of the therapy work associated with TF-CBT will occur between sessions, when parents and children are asked to practice certain skills at home.

- Psychoeducation and Parenting skills
- Relaxation
- Affective modulation
- Cognitive coping and processing
- Trauma narrative
- *In vivo* mastery of trauma reminders
- Conjoint child–parent sessions
- Enhancing future safety and development

SUMMARY

The TF-CBT components are typically provided separately to children and parents in individual sessions, with conjoint child–parent sessions occurring toward the end of therapy. The TF-CBT components build on previously mastered skills such that they should typically be given in the following sequence: psychoeducation and parenting skills, relaxation and affective modulation, cognitive processing, trauma narrative and mastery of trauma reminders, conjoint child–parent sessions, and enhancement of safety and future development. It is important for therapists to be mindful of cultural, religious, and family values when adapting the TF-CBT model for individual children and families, and to be aware of adversities the child and family are experiencing secondary to the traumatic experiences.

CHAPTER 4

The Role of the TF-CBT Therapist

Like any effective therapy, TF-CBT depends first and foremost on a trusting, genuine therapeutic relationship between therapist and the child and parent. It is difficult to capture, in writing, the richness of what really occurs in therapy. In creating a guide for therapists in a particular treatment model, it is necessary to include enough specific technical details so that fidelity to the model is maintained. However, in doing so, the model can end up sounding simplistic or mechanistic, more like a "cookbook" of ingredients and techniques than a creative and interactional therapeutic process. Therapists have often told us that they had thought of cognitive-behavioral therapy as a rigid, formulaic approach, but that experience with the TF-CBT model helped them understand that it is similar to their own therapeutic interventions in the most important way. Specifically, these therapists have mentioned that listening to TF-CBT treatment tapes makes clear to them the centrality of the therapeutic relationship—the therapist's warmth, empathy, insightfulness, creativity, flexibility, and genuine concern for the child and parent. In this chapter we include a detailed discussion of these critical therapeutic elements, which we believe are essential to the success of TF-CBT, or any other child psychotherapy model. We clarify and expand on how these components might be implemented by using the therapist's unique strengths and talents while still maintaining fidelity to the TF-CBT model. We hope that this coverage will convey some of the depth and breadth of the therapeutic process that occurs in the use of this treatment approach.

THE CENTRALITY
OF THE THERAPEUTIC RELATIONSHIP

As noted earlier, traumatized children have often lost trust in others and their former view of the world as a generally fair and safe place. Reestablishing trust often begins with a single reliable, genuine, and caring relationship. Ideally parents provide this connection for their children. However, when a child is traumatized, the parent is often also traumatized, either directly (e.g., if the parent was also exposed to community or domestic violence) or vicariously (e.g., by learning of his/her child being sexually abused). In such instances, parents themselves may be in need of therapeutic assistance before they are able to provide optimal support to their child. Additionally, some children and many adolescents are reticent to turn to parents for support following a traumatic event for fear of further upsetting the parent, especially because they are dependent on their parents in so many ways. Thus the therapist may play a critical role in modeling trustworthiness and providing support to both traumatized children and their parents. Ultimately, TF-CBT aims to assist the parents in regaining their role as the primary therapeutic resource and support for their children.

Therapists sometimes get caught up in completing all the specific "tasks" included in a particular treatment component, to the detriment of the therapeutic relationship. During each therapy session, the therapist should focus attention on the child or parent, not only listening carefully to his/her words but also noticing the accompanying body language and affect. Practicing reflective listening is a powerful way to convey to children and parents that you are not only hearing exactly what they have said, but that you are comfortable with the words and content. What the child and parent have to communicate is important; the successful implementation of TF-CBT depends on the therapist's ability to accurately and empathically understand the source of the child's fear, anger, avoidance, and other difficulties. TF-CBT components must be tailored to fit the needs of each individual child and parent in order to be optimally successful.

Communicating genuineness is also critical to establishing trust; children are adept at detecting the difference between perfunctory attention and true interest in their feelings, thoughts, and lives. Although therapists differ in their comfort in sharing personal information, all therapists using this model should be "real"—that is, not automatons who are simply teaching a set of skills. Thus the therapist must listen carefully and attentively, respect the perspective of the child and parent even when questioning or challenging certain cognitions or parenting practices, and respond appropriately to both the overt and latent content of what is being communicated. Managing these complex levels requires knowledge and skill that goes far beyond simply knowing the specific components of the TF-CBT model. When the therapist successfully communicates that he/she is genuinely concerned about the child and parent and is striving to truly understand and help the child and parent, this trustworthiness is noted by the child and parent and encourages trust toward the therapist.

THE IMPORTANCE OF THERAPIST JUDGMENT, SKILL, AND CREATIVITY

As noted, although this book presents the TF-CBT components in a specific order, it is not essential that the model be implemented in exactly this order or manner with each child and parent. Clinical judgment may dictate that certain issues take precedence over others. For example, dangerous behaviors need to be addressed promptly, regardless of which component the child is working on in treatment. Ideally, the interventions used would be consistent with the TF-CBT model; that is, assisting the child in identifying specific feelings that precede thoughts of self-harm; use of cognitive processing and problem-solving skills to generate alternative thoughts, feelings, and behaviors to self-injurious ones; eliciting appropriate parental praise for noninjury; and encouraging appropriate behavioral and supportive parental responses to dangerous behavior. However, the exact manner in which these interventions are implemented depends on the therapist's judgment regarding to what the child or parent might be most receptive or responsive. The therapist may sometimes use knowledge of family systems, psychodynamic, and other psychotherapeutic approaches to discern the issues underlying the family's difficulty or resistance in optimally using the TF-CBT interventions.

For example, one parent whose child had been in a motor vehicle accident in which the parent was the driver and the child's friend was killed, consistently undermined the therapist's attempts to teach the child relaxation techniques, stating that these never worked for the parent and would not work for the child either. This parent also expressed, in front of the child, a lack of confidence that the TF-CBT components would be successful and suggested that the therapist was insufficiently experienced to help the child. None of the therapist's attempts to join with the parent or to enlist her support for the treatment was successful until the therapist suggested that the mother's guilty feelings about the accident might make her believe that she did not have the right to get well. At this, the mother was able to cry, then state that she did not deserve to ever be happy again, and that her child's continued symptoms were part of her punishment for causing another child's death. Although the child's trauma remained the focus of treatment, the therapist was able to use TF-CBT interventions to explore and challenge the mother's negative cognitions. The mother, meanwhile, feeling that the therapist understood and did not judge what she (the mother) considered to be the worst parts of herself, became better able to support her child's recovery. This breakthrough would likely not have been possible without the therapist's psychodynamic insight into the true reason for the mother's resistance to treatment.

Clinical judgment and knowledge of child development are also essential in working with children and adolescents of different developmental levels, cultural backgrounds, intellectual and cognitive abilities, and interests. Whereas some children readily comply with the therapist's suggestions to engage in specific activities or games, others may refuse to participate in any of these. In this type of situation, the therapist's flexibility, coupled with a broad repertoire of activities through which the TF-CBT interventions can be implemented, is important to the successful implementation of this model. Knowing when to make a joke or give more choices in response to a child's oppositional behavior, versus when to ignore or set firm limits on it, involves therapist experience and judgment—and sometimes just plain good instincts in working with children. Recognizing when a problematic behavior observed in the therapy session (e.g., refusing to participate in any suggested therapeutic activities) is reflecting anger at loss of control versus fear of confronting traumatic memories versus traumatic detachment is a crucial skill in working with some traumatized children, because the therapist's response might need to be quite different in these different situations. A high level of therapist insight, judgment, and creativity is necessary.

Some families come to sessions with a new crisis every week; addressing each new crisis can potentially undermine the effectiveness of any treatment model because there is no continuity or progression to therapy. The therapist must be skilled at balancing the realistic needs to address the family's problems in daily living, with the need for the child to gain increasing trust, new skills, and mastery over the traumatic experiences that brought him/her to treatment in the first place. Knowledge of community resources, skill in accessing these resources for the benefit of the family, and the ability to focus the family on the tasks at hand without seeming to overlook or dismiss their present concerns, are essential assets for therapists attempting to work successfully with such families. Being truly responsive to the family's practical needs may create a more trusting atmosphere in which to provide trauma-specific interventions. For example, we have often found that requesting alternative school placement or temporary homebound instruction for children who are being threatened at school, or helping parents to access wraparound services for another child in the family who has severe behavioral problems, has engaged families who were initially resistant to implementing any changes suggested in therapy. If the therapist is skilled in eliciting information, knowledgeable about community resources, and efficient in accessing these resources, such interventions take relatively little time and leave the family with enough time and greatly increased motivation to benefit from the TF-CBT interventions that the therapist—now perceived as a highly effective and helpful resource—has to offer.

Crises may also offer "natural" opportunities to encourage the use of coping skills acquired in treatment. In some instances it may be most appropriate for the therapist to utilize a portion of the session to assist clients in applying effective coping skills to address the crisis, then returning to trauma-focused work for the remainder of the session. This treatment rhythm may be particularly important with highly avoidant adolescents who present with weekly crises as a way to avoid the sometimes distressing aspects of trauma-focused treatment. Thus the therapist's skills, knowledge, judgment, and creativity, as applied to children, families, child development, traumatology, and child psychotherapy, are all important assets in the optimal implementation of TF-CBT.

THERAPIST QUALIFICATIONS AND TRAINING

Given the complexities of working with children who have been traumatized and their families, we strongly recommend that this treatment manual only be implemented by therapists who have received training in child development and who are experienced in assessing and treating a wide range of different child psychiatric disorders. Additionally, therapists should have prior training and supervision in providing a variety of treatment approaches to children and their families, including insight-oriented/psychodynamic, family systems, interpersonal, cognitive-behavioral, and/or play therapies. Finally, therapists should have access to supervisors and/or consultants who have received intensive training in, and have implemented, the TF-CBT treatment model.

Based on our experience of training hundreds of therapists in the TF-CBT model, we recommend the following training for therapists wishing to use this treatment model.

• Initial introductory training in the treatment model is typically offered in a 1- to 3-day training experience provided by the authors or their designated trainers. Additionally, a 6-hour videotaped training is available. Following are additional training opportunities to further support clinical skill development in TF-CBT.

• Alternatively, web-based training in the TF-CBT model is available at www.musc.edu/tfcbt at the time of this writing. This web-based learning course includes streaming demonstrations, videos, cultural considerations, and examples of how to address complex situations for each TF-CBT component. Additionally, once practitioners register for the course, they can return to it as often as they like for review.

• Ongoing expert consultation is suggested for implementing this treatment model with multiproblem children and families, as well as for professionals who wish to supervise others in the TF-CBT model. We have provided this type of ongoing consultation to over 100 therapists throughout the United States, and are currently developing a TF-CBT "Train the Trainers" program to expand this effort.

• Advanced training in implementing TF-CBT is also recommended to further enhance clinical skill development. This training, along with ongoing case-specific consultation, is also recommended for optimal supervision of other therapists in the use of this model.

TROUBLESHOOTING

You mentioned families who bring in crises every week? What are some ways to address this problem?

This is one of the most frequent questions we get asked. The therapist should talk directly with the parent about the importance of doing trauma-focused therapy with the child and parent in order to address the child's trauma symptoms. It will be important to remind the parent of these symptoms, as assessed by the UCLA PTSD Index for DSM-IV (Pynoos, Rodriguez, et al., 1998) or other instruments completed by the child and parent during the evaluation to document the need for trauma-specific interventions. Then the therapist can offer several alternatives to address the ongoing crises. It is essential to acknowledge these openly, because doing so communicates to the parent, "I recognize the importance of your concerns; these are troublesome, real problems in your life that merit attention right now." Here are some options:

1. Provide another therapeutic alternative to address these crises (e.g., child's severe behavior problems): wraparound services, family-based treatment, mobile crisis, in-home services, group therapy, case management, etc.

2. Devote half of each session to these issues, with the agreement that the other half will be spent on trauma-focused therapy.

3. Agree to set aside trauma issues for a specified treatment period (e.g., 5 weeks) and to focus exclusively on behavioral/family stabilization for that period. Establish specific goals for that time period and if they are attained, start the TF-CBT. If not, consider the possibility that the family is not ready to commit to trauma-focused work and that it would be better to delay this work until the family is more stable or until ancillary services are available.

What if parents are unwilling to bring children to regular treatment appointments? We have many families who attend irregularly. Can this model be used?

We believe that regular attendance is necessary for any treatment to be effective for traumatized children. Because TF-CBT builds on previously mastered components as well as a trusting, therapeutic relationship, it is doubly important for families to come to therapy on a regular basis. We explain this point to parents at the start of treatment, adding that treatment may take as little as 10–12 weeks if they attend regularly. We sometimes ask families to agree to a treatment contract stating that they will come only for that many sessions, after which time they will reassess their child's progress together and then decide whether further treatment is needed. Knowing they will have the option to terminate at that point allows many families to make a short-term commitment to treatment that they might not otherwise make.

What do you do about frequently missed appointments?

We explain to parents that their children will not be able to remember what they learned in previous sessions and that treatment cannot be as helpful as it should be. Then we usually suggest that this may not be the right time for them to come to therapy and offer them an "out" from treatment. Many families respond by attending regularly from that point on, whereas others acknowledge that they cannot commit to treatment at this time.

What if the parent seems to need more help with his/her own trauma issues and tries to make treatment about him/her instead of about the child?

In these situations we try to focus on the following:

1. Help parent refocus on the child's needs by carefully reviewing the treatment goals while maintaining the structure and focus of sessions to achieve these goals.

2. Point out to the parent that his/her child does not have to experience the same difficulties that he/she has (and point out the ways he/she, the parent, has protected the child from this fate so far).

3. Help the parent maintain a present-day focus on how to help the child with current symptoms in the context of the TF-CBT treatment model.

4. Focus on positive child–parent interactions and ways to optimize these.

5. Optimize support to the parent in every possible way.

6. When appropriate, refer the parent for his/her own individual therapy. Given the time commitment and investment associated with participating in therapy, for some parents it may be best to complete the course of therapy for their child before entering into treatment for themselves. However, it is important to carefully consider the timing of such a referral. Other parents may be receptive and may greatly benefit from a referral for individual therapy soon after a trusting therapeutic relationship has been established. We have found some parents to have such severe personal trauma histories and/or such significant personality issues of their own that opening up these issues would not be feasible or productive in a short-term, child-centered treatment approach.

PART II

TRAUMA-FOCUSED
COMPONENTS

Introduction to
the TF-CBT Components

As noted earlier, the TF-CBT components are psychoeducation, parenting skills, relaxation, affective modulation, cognitive coping and processing, trauma narrative, *in vivo* mastery of trauma reminders, conjoint child–parent sessions, and enhancing future safety and development. These components are summarized by the PRACTICE acronym. The TF-CBT model has been tested under conditions that applied the components generally in this order. It is therefore important for therapists to understand that the efficacy of the TF-CBT model is known only in relation to the use of all of the components in the order they are introduced in this manual. The order of the components is also based on a logical sequence of skill building. Certain skills are learned and consolidated before others that depend on the previously learned skills are introduced. For example, affective modulation and relaxation are early TF-CBT components that are ideally mastered in the first few treatment sessions. Cognitive coping is introduced after affective modulation because it relies on the child's and parent's ability to differentiate feelings from thoughts. Having already learned to identify and manage a variety of feelings in the early affective modulation component, the child and parent will be better prepared to address the more complex task of integrating the connections among these feelings with a variety of thoughts and behaviors. Similarly, parenting skills are taught early in treatment to enhance the parent's ability to encourage positive child behaviors and provide needed support to the child as more challenging trauma-focused parts of treatment are addressed later. In addition, this skill-building parenting component aims to enhance the parent's ability to deal with any problematic behaviors.

Consolidating all of these early coping skills for the child and parent—affective modulation, relaxation, and cognitive coping, and parenting skills for the parent—helps to optimize the positive outcome of the trauma narrative and *in vivo* exposure components of treatment. We have told trainees, "The time to learn to tread water is not when you are in the middle of the ocean." Similarly, the optimal time to learn stress management skills is not in the middle of creating a trauma narrative but long before you start one. This is the rationale for providing the TF-CBT components in the sequence they are introduced in this book, and we believe that they should be provided to children in this order in most cases. However, therapists might return to previously learned components to review them at times when children or parents appear to need a review or reinforcement of those components. This practice is certainly consistent with the TF-CBT model and something we have done many times. Another exception might be conducting conjoint child–parent sessions earlier in treatment to address important issues that need to be faced as a family. This practice would also be consistent with the TF-CBT model, as long as the focus of the session was on a TF-CBT component appropriate for that stage of treatment (e.g., if therapy had progressed to the cognitive-processing component, then the joint sessions should focus on components up to that point, not suddenly skip ahead to the trauma narrative or *in vivo* mastery). Additionally, flexibility should be used in determining how many sessions each individual child and family needs in mastering each component. For example, some children with "complex trauma" may need many sessions to master affective modulation before moving on to cognitive coping.

To summarize, the TF-CBT components should generally be provided in the order they are introduced in this book, and all of the TF-CBT components should be provided to all children who are receiving the treatment model. Exceptions include returning to previously covered components for review and incorporating joint child–parent sessions or family sessions at any time if clinically indicated.

Psychoeducation

Psychoeducation is one of the major components of TF-CBT. Although it is introduced at the outset of treatment, psychoeducation continues throughout the therapy process with both the child and caretaker. The primary goals of psychoeducation are to normalize both the child's and parent's response to the traumatic events and to reinforce accurate cognitions about what occurred. These goals are critical, given the often painful and confusing feelings that a child and parent experience in the aftermath of a trauma.

Psychoeducation actually begins at the initial intake phone call. As the caretaker describes the traumatic event, the child's reactions to it, and his/her own responses, the intake worker should be supportive and try to normalize both the child's and parent's responses. In this regard, it is very comforting for a parent to learn that his/her child's responses following a traumatic event are not unusual, even though the child may be behaving in ways that are not typical for him/her.

When the parent learns that clinicians at our centers have treated many children who have experienced the same trauma as their child and that most children "get better," these are words of hope that almost always provide some sense of emotional relief. It is important to mention that psychoeducation continues during the assessment with the same goals of normalizing the child's and parent's responses to the traumatic event and reinforcing accurate cognitions.

The initial step is to provide general information to both the child and parent about the traumatic event. This information can include the frequency of the specific trauma that the child has experienced, who typically experiences it, and what causes it. For example, with respect to sexual abuse, we provide information sheets to both the child and parent that include such information as how many children are sexually abused by the age of 18, what are the different types of sexual abuse, who molests children, and why many children do not tell others about the sexual abuse. These information sheets can dispel many myths that the child and parent have about sexual abuse and its consequences. In a similar way, we try to provide general information about whatever trauma a child has experienced. When the child and parent learn "facts" about the effects of witnessing domestic violence or being a victim of school or community violence, etc., misinformation is dispelled and child and parent learn that many other families have encountered a similar terrifying or tragic event and that this particular family is not alone with regard to the difficult challenges that they now face. Sample information sheets are included in Appendix 1.

The next step in psychoeducation is to provide information about common emotional and behavioral responses to the traumatic event that the child has experienced. Any available empirical information bearing on this issue is shared with both the child and parent. Scientific information that documents common reactions to a specific type of trauma provides significant emotional validation for both the child and parent, who learn that their responses are not so unusual. In addition, clinicians typically have seen other children who have experienced the same traumatic event and can provide firsthand feedback to both the child and parent that their emotional and behavioral reactions are more the norm than the exception. This feedback is also highly validating for both the child and parent.

Another way to provide information about common reactions is to utilize children's books that describe what a child may experience after a traumatic event. Many of these types of books have been written by professionals who have learned about common reactions to trauma because of their direct clinical experience. Even more compelling may be children's books written by older adolescents or adults who survived a traumatic event during childhood and are now telling their "story." These books convey to children that they are not alone in what they have experienced, that their feelings are expected, given what occurred, and that there are ways to deal with their painful feelings that result in personal growth and healing.

Providing specific information about the child's diagnosis is another aspect of psychoeducation. Although this experience can be frightening for both the child and parent (i.e., what parent wants to hear that his/her child has a diagnosable disorder?), it can also turn out to be quite helpful if the clinician provides the diagnostic information in a straightforward manner devoid of excessive clinical terminology. For example, if a child has PTSD, the reexperiencing symptoms can be described as painful reminders of the trauma and the avoidant symptoms as a way for the child to try to obtain relief from this emotional pain. For the hyperarousal symptoms (e.g., distractibility, difficulty sleeping, irritability), the child and parent can be told that these are ways that the brain and/or body indicate that the traumatic event has overwhelmed the child's physical ability to cope. Children and parents appreciate a straightforward explanation that can be easily comprehended, and they are more likely to form a therapeutic connection with a clinician whom they can see as down-to-earth and "real."

In addition to providing information about symptoms and diagnosis, this part of psychoeducation includes giving descriptions of available treatments. In this regard, it is always reassuring for children and parents to learn that TF-CBT has strong empirical support and that the majority of children who receive treatment with this model experience a significant reduction in symptomatology and develop solid coping skills. It is worth noting that parents, in particular, are often very worried that their child will never overcome the effects of the trauma. Informing them that our research has demonstrated that even children with serious symptoms or multiple traumas improve after treatment conveys a sense of hope and confidence and increases the likelihood that the family will follow through with treatment recommendations.

A final and often unrecognized aspect of psychoeducation is to provide strategies to the child and parent to manage current symptoms. This step is important for at least three reasons. First, symptomatic relief is, of course, an end unto itself. For example, a child with PTSD who is experiencing significant sleep disruption may have trouble concentrating at school or may be more prone to angry outbursts or irritability at home. Moreover, when a child's sleep is disrupted, it is quite likely that the parent's sleep will become disrupted as well. Accordingly, everyone in the family benefits when behavioral or other strategies are used to address this common problem.

A second reason to manage current symptoms is because doing so conveys to the child and (especially) the parent that their concerns are understood and respected. If a parent tells the clinician that the child's sleep difficulties have disrupted the entire family but the clinician ignores this plea for help or suggests that this problem will be addressed many weeks into treatment, the parent is likely to feel invalidated, as if what they deem important will not be a priority. In TF-CBT, the child's/parent's concerns are taken seriously, and strategies are developed right from the outset of treatment to address them. From our perspective, this approach conveys the true spirit of collaboration between the therapist and child/parent that is at the heart of the TF-CBT model.

Finally, successfully managing current symptoms early in treatment breeds confidence in the therapist and the TF-CBT model for both the child and parent. Hope is important when families encounter difficult challenges after a traumatic event. And nothing breeds hope like success. Additionally, the increased trust in the therapist because of these early improvements will make it more likely that the child/parent can be engaged in subsequent aspects of treatment that may be more anxiety provoking (e.g., creating the trauma narrative).

Although it is crucial that psychoeducation strategies be used at the beginning of treatment, they can also be utilized frequently throughout the treatment process. For example, the therapist may inform the parent and/or child that some resistance to creating a trauma narrative is not unusual in children. Moreover, it can be useful to predict for the parent(s) that sometimes children exhibit increased avoidance and/or a mild exacerbation of symptoms when beginning the trauma narrative work. If these behaviors occur, parents are asked to share their observations with the therapist and to respond to their children's avoidance with encouragement and a demonstration of their own commitment to attending therapy. In addition, the therapist can indicate to a parent that in his/her clinical practice he/she has often observed the cognitive distortions (e.g., self-blame; unrealistic sense of threat in the world) that the parent is currently experiencing. Again, psychoeducation in either instance normalizes the child's or parent's responses, which results in emotional validation, a sense of increased acceptance, and a greater likelihood of cooperation during the treatment process.

PSYCHOEDUCATION ABOUT THE TF-CBT MODEL OF TREATMENT

It is important for the therapist to spend a few minutes in the initial session orienting the parent to the TF-CBT model. This orientation consists of explaining the philosophy of using this approach and should include the following elements:

- The child is having significant PTSD or other trauma-related symptoms.
- Clinical experience as well as research suggests that these PTSD and other trauma-related symptoms need to be addressed as early as possible to prevent long-term difficulties.
- Briefly review the PTSD and other trauma-related symptoms the child is experiencing, based on the clinical assessment that has been completed prior to treatment initiation.
- Talking directly about the trauma is important in resolving these difficulties and integrating the experience into the child's life in an optimal way.
- This component will be implemented in a gradual, supportive manner so that the child will be able to tolerate the discomfort associated with such discussion; furthermore, it will typically not be initiated until the child has learned some skills to help him/her cope with the discomfort.
- The therapist will work in collaboration with the parent throughout treatment, and the therapist welcomes the parent's suggestions at any time.
- People of different religions, ethnicities, and cultures have different ways of expressing and dealing with trauma responses; the therapist is eager to learn from the child and parent the traditions and rituals of their culture, religion, and family and will remain respectful of these in the treatment process.

PSYCHOEDUCATION FOR CHILDREN EXPERIENCING TRAUMATIC GRIEF

Children who have experienced a trauma that resulted in the death of a loved one may need additional psychoeducational information. For example, depending on the cause of death, it may be important to acknowledge intentionality if the death was due to terrorism or intentional (as opposed to random) homicide. Assimilating information about why people commit these acts is difficult even for adults, and parents (or perhaps the family's religious leader) might be consulted with regard to how this might be explained to the child in a manner that is consistent with the family's beliefs and the child's developmental capacities. Additional information about death and mourning are provided in the grief-focused psychoeducation component.

TROUBLESHOOTING

What if the child has multiple comorbid conditions? Won't providing psychoeducation about these problems lead to pessimism rather than optimism about the child's future?

The therapist should always be as honest as possible about the child's difficulties, while still emphasizing the positive aspects of the child's and family's circumstances. Accurately identifying the child's comorbid conditions can actually be a relief to parents who might have spent many years wondering what has been the cause of the child's many problems, which may have predated the traumatic events that brought the child to treatment. Several excellent resources are available for parents whose children have comorbid conditions such as ADHD (e.g., *Taking Charge of ADHD: The Complete, Authoritative Guide for Parents*, Revised Edition, by Russell Barkley) or bipolar disorder (e.g., *New Hope for Children and Teens with Bipolar Disorder: Your Friendly, Authoritative Guide to the Latest in Traditional and Complementary Solutions*, by Boris Birmaher). We believe that providing psychoeducation about possible preexisting or coexisting psychiatric conditions can decrease the guilt, burden, and frustration that many families experience when they don't understand why their child is not doing well. Helping families get the help that is available for these conditions gives them hope that things can get better.

Diagnosing a comorbid condition in the face of acute or ongoing traumatic exposure can be very difficult, so the therapist should be clear in discussing different possibilities in this regard. Providing information about a variety of differential diagnostic possibilities, along with a plan for how each of these possibilities will be evaluated, is very helpful to families. For some disorders, specific evaluations or information can be obtained while trauma-focused treatment is being provided (e.g., testing for learning disabilities can be performed or teacher ratings can be obtained for suspected ADHD). Sometimes it is better to take a "wait-and-see" approach, for example, suggesting that the child's difficulties may resolve with trauma-focused treatment and that trauma-focused psychotherapy be tried initially. If over a certain period of time it becomes clear that the child's difficulties are not responding to trauma-focused interventions alone, they may need to be supplemented or replaced by other types of psychotherapy and/or medication. It is reasonable to acknowledge that you don't have all the answers to the child's problems when the child presents with a complex clinical picture, and reasonable parents will understand this difficulty and appreciate your honesty.

What if a parent asks a question that you don't think is appropriate to answer in front of the child?

The therapist should feel free to define some information as being for "adults only" or "for kids and parents to share." Children are used to such boundaries (or should be), and parents should be able to set such limits on their children listening to adult conversations. The therapist can then meet privately with the parent to share "adult only" information and use this time to model for the parent how and why certain questions might be inappropriate to ask in front of the child.

How can therapists ascertain how much information is "too much" for parents to hear in one session?

There is often a temptation to provide parents with all of the psychoeducation available in the first session in the hope that this information will help them feel better about their child's situation. However, there is a risk that some families will feel overwhelmed by all this information. It may be helpful to provide some educational information during a treatment session, while also providing written material (e.g., brief information sheets) to be reviewed at home. In terms of time spent during the session, the therapist should gauge the parent's response whether too much information is being provided. Every so often, ask whether the parent has any questions. If there are no questions, it may be time to stop giving information because the parent may be overloaded for the time being. Remember that psychoeducation can continue throughout the course of treatment.

What if children or parents ask about your personal trauma history? Do you tell them the truth in this regard?

This is a personal decision. There may be both benefits and risks associated with telling or not telling your patients information about your personal trauma history, particularly with regard to certain types of trauma such as sexual abuse, which is associated with a great deal of emotional meaning. It is important to remember that the meaning it has to you, as a therapist, to tell this to a patient may be quite different than it has to your patients. If you do share such information, it is important to be clear in your own mind about your reasons for doing this while also minimizing the sharing of details that might be troubling or distracting for some children and parents.

Ideally, you would be sharing your personal trauma experience with your patient or patient's parent in order to convey an increased sense of understanding and empathy regarding what they have experienced.

While it is true that many families may have greater trust in a personal trauma survivor who understands the family's personal agony and pain, the trade-off is that the therapist has to give up his or her privacy regarding this history. If the family has appropriate boundaries, this loss of privacy is not likely to become problematic. But if a family member has difficulties maintaining boundaries, the therapist may regret revealing this personal information as family members may misinterpret the intention of the therapist's disclosure.

We have also seen occasional situations in which, far from increasing therapists' credibility when they have disclosed their personal trauma histories, family members have instead become offended or dismissive, assuming these therapists were only treating traumatized children in order to work out their own unresolved personal issues from their trauma experiences. Alternatively, such family members might become over-solicitous, offering concerned comments (e.g., "Oh, I'm so sorry," "Are you okay hearing about this again?" "This must trigger all kinds of sad memories for you."). When children or parents feel they have to console or question you about your own emotional well-being, self-disclosure has not served a positive therapeutic purpose for your patients.

What if the child does not seem interested in reading the information sheet?

We have found that children respond particularly well to psychoeducation when information is presented in the context of a question-and-answer game. Therapists can pose the questions on the information sheets, allowing children to receive points and/or praise for what they know, while also providing a mechanism for the therapist to offer additional information and/or identify and correct any misconceptions the child may have.

Parenting Skills

In the face of a child's experiencing a severely traumatic life event, even the most competent parent may have difficulty in parenting effectively. As we have noted before, this challenge creates added barriers to the healing process because maintaining normal routines and consistency in rules and expectations in the face of stress promotes adaptive functioning in children as well as adults. For parents who did not have optimal parenting skills prior to the traumatic event, gaining these skills may be even more crucial in optimizing the child's outcome. These skills are particularly needed when children respond to traumatization with aggression, angry outbursts, and other negative behaviors (AACAP, 1998). The parenting skills included in TF-CBT, although basic and easy to learn, have been found to have a great impact on parenting abilities in parents of children experiencing behavioral problems in response to trauma such as sexual abuse (Deblinger et al., 1996; Cohen & Mannarino, 1996a) and multiple traumas (Cohen, Deblinger, et al., 2004), as well as children with primary behavioral problems. These skills include the use of praise, selective attention, effective time-out procedures, and contingency reinforcement schedules (behavior charts). We typically introduce these parental skills along with psychoeducation in the first few treatment sessions. These skills are especially relevant for children who are having behavioral problems, but they are also helpful for children who are not exhibiting behavioral difficulties. Emphasizing the positive power of praise, for example, early in treatment can have a very powerful impact on the child–parent relationship.

PRAISE

Most people thrive upon praise or positive attention. Most parents believe that they praise their children frequently and consistently, but in fact many parents devote more time to correcting or criticizing their children for negative behaviors than to praising them for positive behaviors. The therapist should start by asking the parent what his/her child does right or well or what the parent is most proud of the child for doing. Then the therapist should ask the parent how often he/she verbally praises the child for these behaviors. Upon reflection, the parent may realize that these positive behaviors are taken for granted and therefore not often noticed or singled out for verbal comment. As a consequence, these behaviors may not occur as frequently as desired. The therapist should instruct the parent to focus on actively praising the child for positive behaviors in the coming week and note the effect of this praise on the child's mood and subsequent behavior.

As part of this instruction, the therapist should specify how to effectively give praise. This instruction includes the following:

- Praise a specific behavior (e.g., say "I like how you took out the garbage the first time I asked.") rather than providing global praise (e.g., "You're a great kid."). This type of praise will allow the child to more readily identify the behavior with which you are pleased. Children crave praise, and the better they understand how to get it, the more you will see the positive behaviors.
- Provide praise as soon as possible after the behavior has occurred.
- Be consistent; praise the behavior each time it occurs (at least, at first).
- Do not qualify your praise. For example, do not say "I'm so glad you took out the garbage when I asked. Why can't you listen like that more often?" This phrasing turns the intended praise into a criticism of the child.
- Provide praise with the same level of intensity that you would provide criticism. Many parents praise faintly ("nice job"), but criticize loudly, with great emotional intensity ("How could you *do* a thing like this?!!!"). If a child is trying to get intense, focused attention from the parent and can only get it through negative behaviors, the negative behaviors will continue.

Having parents role-play with the therapist various scenarios where they praise their child may help the therapist correct in the session any errors the parents may be making in their attempts to praise. As noted above, a common error parents make that undermines the power of praise involves the addition of a negative tag following the praise: "You cleaned your room so nicely" is a great example of praise, until the parent adds the negative tag, "Why don't you keep your room like this all the time?"

Some parents may have difficulty identifying any praiseworthy behavior in their child. Childhood PTSD is sometimes manifested by irritable mood and angry outbursts (APA, 2000), and parents may be focused, understandably, on these behaviors. The therapist should encourage such parents to "catch your child being good," or at least catch times when the child is exhibiting no overtly negative behaviors, and offer praise (e.g., "It's so nice to sit here with you watching TV so peacefully."). When children respond to such comments with sullen responses ("just leave me alone"), the parent has the perfect opportunity to practice active ignoring, as described below.

Parents are also encouraged to listen actively and participate with children when they engage in healthy conversation and/or positive behaviors. Too often parents inadvertently attend to negative child behaviors more than to positive behaviors. Examining the pattern of child–parent interactions and helping parents increase their efforts to attend to positive behaviors via praise, listening, and participating with their children can dramatically reverse the escalation of problem behaviors.

SELECTIVE ATTENTION

When a parent consciously makes a decision to not react to certain negative behaviors the child exhibits, he/she is using selective attention. This approach is based on the idea that children want focused, emotionally intense attention from their parents and others, and that they will continue to exhibit behaviors that get this type of attention, even if the attention takes a negative form (e.g., yelling from the parent). Without realizing it, parents often attend and respond more to misbehavior in their children than to good behavior. Thus they are inadvertently reinforcing (i.e., rewarding through attention) the very negative behaviors they want to discourage. In order to reinforce *desired* behaviors, the parent must learn to praise these good behaviors and selectively ignore most negative ones. Of course, the parent cannot and should not ignore overtly dangerous behaviors (discussed below). Examples of behaviors to which parents often respond negatively but which would be better selectively ignored include the following:

- Temper tantrums or angry verbalizations directed at the parent
- Making nasty faces, rolling eyes, smirking at parent
- Mocking, taunting, mimicking the parent
- Provocative comments meant to be intentionally annoying

The therapist should point out to the parent that such behaviors, although unpleasant, are not harmful and are most often the child's effort to "get the parent's goat," that is, to provoke a negative response. If the negative responses are no longer forthcoming, the behaviors eventually stop. The parent should practice walking away calmly, without commenting on such behaviors, and busy him/herself with another activity in another part of the room or in a different room from the child. The therapist can add that this technique may result in an escalation to even more provocative behaviors (known as an "extinction burst") that should be taken as a sign that the parent is effectively withdrawing his/her negative attention. If the parent can continue to withhold his/her attention through this period of escalation, the problem behavior is very likely to cease. Unfortunately, parents should be warned that if they attend to the behavior at the height of its intensity, the child will learn that he/she needs to get really loud to regain his/her parents' negative attention. If a parent feels that he/she will be unable to maintain a stance of selective inattention throughout such an escalation, then the parent should plan to use a time-out. However, above all, the parent should maintain a calm, dispassionate, controlled demeanor to avoid giving the child the reinforcing negative attention he/she is seeking. Equally important, the next moment the child is behaving well, the parent should give positive attention (praise) for this behavior. An added benefit of selective inattention is that the parent saves him/herself from emotional distress by remaining calm and unflustered despite the child's negative behaviors.

TIME-OUT

The purposes of the time-out procedure are to (1) interrupt the child's negative behaviors and thus allow him/her to regain emotional and behavioral control; and (2) to deprive the child of the opportunity to receive any type of attention. Ideally, the parent should explain the time-out procedure to the child before the first time it is used, stating that if the child does not comply with the parent's request to stop a particular behavior, the parent will place the child in time out. Time-outs should be located in the quietest, least stimulating room available, and should only last 1 minute for every year of age (for example, a 7-year-old should have a 7-minute time-out). Before initiating the time-out procedure, the parent should calmly ask the child to stop the undesired behavior, specifying the undesired behavior exactly (e.g., "Please stop kicking the door," rather than "BEHAVE!"). If the behavior continues, the parent may remind the child once that he/she will go to time-out if the behavior does not stop. If the child does not stop, the parent should escort the child to the designated time-out area, without any further comment, and with a calm, dispassionate demeanor. The parent should refrain from responding to the child's verbalizations or further negative behaviors. The timer should be set when the child has stopped screaming, banging on the walls, etc., in the time-out room. Once the time has elapsed, the parent should retrieve the child from time-out and proceed with normal activities. If the child is now acting in an appropriate manner, the parent should interact positively with the child, giving positive attention and refraining from showing annoyance or anger about the previous behavior problems. In this way the child learns that good behavior leads to positive parental attention, whereas problem behavior leads to time-out (i.e., no attention). Parents who are able to implement time-out consistently often see rapid behavioral improvements in their children and feel more competent about their own parenting skills because they are not losing control, yelling, hitting, or engaging in other angry parenting responses. More persistent behavioral problems may be addressed through the use of contingency reinforcement programs, which are briefly described below.

CONTINGENCY REINFORCEMENT PROGRAMS

Contingency reinforcement programs—that is, the utilization of behavior charts—are useful for decreasing unwanted behaviors and/or for increasing desired behaviors in many children. This intervention is described in great detail elsewhere (Bloomquist, 2006), and therapists are referred there for specific instructions. Briefly, behavior charts should adhere to the following guidelines:

- Select only one behavior at a time to target for change.
- Discuss with the child exactly how to earn a star on the chart (e.g., "Every day that you cooperate in the morning and get to school on time, you will get a star.").
- Involve the child in decisions about what the reward will be (e.g., "I will go to a movie alone with Mom on Sunday if I have gotten five stars between Monday and Saturday.").

- Add up stars and give rewards at least weekly.
- Give stars and rewards consistently.

If the child is exhibiting significant behavioral problems, the therapist should attempt to assess whether these are manifestations of the child's PTSD symptoms or were present before the traumatic event. If the therapist finds that the behavioral problems are becoming the main focus of treatment, referral for ancillary treatment to address those problems may be advisable. In fact, the parent may have brought the child for treatment because of these behavioral problems rather than to address trauma issues, and if the therapist fails to address these in some manner, the parent will likely be dissatisfied and less likely to attend or comply with other aspects of the treatment.

In families where the children's trauma resulted in the death of a parent or sibling, even the most competent parents may experience difficulty in implementing optimal parenting practices. This difficulty may result from (1) their own traumatic stress or grief reactions, (2) feeling that they do not want to inflict any more pain on the child by disciplining him/her now (overpermissiveness), or (3) other misguided attempts to lessen the child's suffering. However, maintaining normal routines and consistency in rules and expectations in the face of the stress of traumatic grief promotes adaptive functioning for children even in these trying circumstances. Providing parents with this information may be helpful. Gaining these skills may be even more crucial to optimizing the child's outcome for parents who did not have optimal parenting skills prior to the death. Issues that accompany suddenly becoming a single parent are addressed in greater detail in Part III of this book.

Finally, parents often benefit from reading supplemental material on parenting. Parenting books that we have utilized and recommend for use in this manner are included in Appendix 2. Specific chapters can be assigned as homework, depending on the family's areas of difficulties.

TROUBLESHOOTING

What do you tell a parent who insists her child "will not take a 'time-out'?"

Often this parent is not consistently implementing the time-out procedure. Asking the child to go to time-out rather than *telling* him/her to go or taking him/her conveys ambivalence about implementing the time-out. It is important to be emphatic about the seriousness of the time-out rule. Children should understand that when they are instructed to go to time-out, they will not be allowed to have any privileges (e.g., TV, computer, phone) until the time-out is completed. Every request a child makes following a time-out instruction (e.g., "Can I watch TV?") should be answered in a monotone, "broken-record" retort: "not until you do your time-out." A time-out room that contains toys, games, TVs, or other fun activities is overstimulating and does not provide the child with the atmosphere to regain control. If the parent is "unable" to take the child to a time-out location without a physical confrontation, the parent instead can remove him/herself to another room (effectively giving him/herself a time-out), thereby depriving the child of his/her attention for the designated time period. If nothing else, this tactic will allow the parent some time to destress from the child's misbehavior.

Some parents are so harsh and critical with their young children. How can I encourage parents to praise their kids more?

Some parents of traumatized children were traumatized themselves as children and never learned to be nurturing parents. Modeling praising behavior by noticing and remarking on the parents' positive actions may be helpful in this regard (in effect, "catch them" being good parents). Praise the smallest maternal gesture you observe on these mothers' parts (e.g., helping the child remove a coat), remark on the child's good behavior as a positive reflection on her parenting skills, etc. We have repeatedly seen these parents respond remarkably positively to praise; they have gotten so little of it in their own lives that it carries a highly positive valence.

In some cultures, it is considered disrespectful for children to stick out their tongues, roll their eyes, etc., and parents would never tolerate or ignore these behaviors. How can you encourage these parents to use selective attention?

Point out to parents that by yelling at children for "disrespecting them," they are reinforcing the very behavior they want to stop. It is not a matter of totally ignoring unacceptable, disrespectful behaviors; it is more a matter of rebalancing the amount of attention paid to those behaviors relative to more appropriate behaviors. These parents may be ignoring 10 minutes of reasonably OK behavior, then yelling when they spot the unwanted behaviors. The goal is to reverse the balance of attention so that the parent is giving much more praise and attention to the 10 minutes of decent behavior and withdrawing attention and praise when the bad behavior happens. The parent may be surprised to see that the bad behavior does not happen even when attention is given to positive interactions. The mother turning away, withdrawing, and quietly saying, "I don't like that behavior" is a very potent punishment when the child has been getting lots of praise and attention up to that point.

For very young children, doesn't selective inattention, or ignoring, give a message of rejection that could be more emotionally damaging?

Of course these parenting skills must be tailored to be age appropriate. The parent should not ignore a very young child (2–3 years old) by leaving to go to another room, because doing so could be dangerous and hurtful. The parent and therapist should work together to design an appropriate way to withdraw attention from the child's negative behavior; it could be as simple as looking away from the child, explaining to the child that that was not a nice thing to do, that it hurt Mommy's feelings, or that it was not a safe behavior. Most importantly, selective inattention is not effective if it is not combined with efforts to provide more positive parental attention, particularly for prosocial behaviors that can replace the problem behavior (e.g., minimizing attention to whining while increasing praise to polite requests or efforts to use a pleasant tone of voice). All behavioral interventions must be individualized to fit the child and parent being treated.

TRAUMA-FOCUSED COMPONENT 3

Relaxation

Relaxation techniques are helpful in reducing the physiological manifestation of stress and PTSD, such as increased adrenergic tone (higher resting heartbeat and faster heart rate in response to stress), increased startle response, hypervigilance, agitation, difficulty sleeping, restlessness and irritability, and anger/rage reactions. These manifestations may be especially problematic when the child experiences traumatic reminders and may occur at some points when the child is creating the trauma narrative. For this reason, we typically teach and practice relaxation techniques prior to having the child create the trauma narrative or engage in other gradual exposure exercises.

First it may be helpful to explain to children the difference between normal and traumatic stress reactions. (More information about how our bodies react to stress is included in Appendix 1 in the Relaxation Handout.)

"All people are born with ways of responding to stress that affect their bodies. When any person experiences a scary event, it is natural to feel afraid and to have specific body reactions that occur in response to chemicals in our brains. Some of these body reactions include:

- Quick, shallow breathing/shortness of breath
- Muscle tension
- Anxious feelings, feeling like we are on "high alert"

and may also include:

- Headaches, dizziness, lightheadedness
- Stomachaches, nausea
- Skin rashes, itching, other irritation

Usually when the danger goes away, these body reactions resolve and our hearts, breathing, etc., go back to how they were before the danger. When children experience traumatic events, however, their bodies may remain on high alert. In this state, any other frightening events, thoughts, or reminders may trigger even more body reactions, leading to an ongoing state of tension and anxiety, both in body and feelings. The good news is that we can do things to reverse this process so that you can return to being calm and relaxed."

The therapist can then instruct the child in the use of the following relaxation strategies and practice these in the session.

FOCUSED BREATHING/MINDFULNESS/MEDITATION

Focused breathing, mindfulness, and meditation are related practices that produce a "relaxation response" (Benson, 1975). The relaxation response has been shown to reverse the adverse physiological and psychological impact of stress in adults and children (Kabat-Zinn, 1990). The following techniques have been adapted for children of different ages. The therapist instructs the child to close his/her eyes and to breathe in deeply so that the lower abdomen protrudes during inhalation and recedes during exhalation. (This is the opposite of chest breathing, where the chest expands and the abdomen is pulled in during inhalation.) Younger children can be assisted in producing this belly breathing by lying on the floor and putting a small book or stuffed animal on their lower abdomen; when this object rises during inhalation, they are doing belly breathing correctly. Once the child has mastered the knack of belly breathing, the therapist instructs the child to slowly count to five while breathing in, and then to exhale slowly through the mouth during another five-count period. Many children will breathe in slowly but exhale quickly unless specifically instructed in this manner. Some children, particularly those who have experienced sexual abuse, may feel too vulnerable to lie on the floor (i.e., this position may be a trauma reminder); in such instances, it may be preferable to practice this skill in a sitting position with eyes open.

Perhaps the most difficult element of focused breathing or mindfulness is that of directed attention, which younger children may not be able to understand. The relaxation response is thought to come at least in part from "quieting" one's thoughts and consistently refocusing on one's breathing rather than being distracted either by external objects/events or internal thoughts or feelings. By directing all of one's attention to the act of breathing, one simultaneously experiences profound relaxation (loss of tension) and focused awareness. The therapist should instruct the older child or adolescent to be aware of any thoughts that arise during the breathing exercise and to redirect his/her attention back to the moving in and out of air through the body as soon as he/she becomes aware of such a thought. The goal is not to judge, reject, or focus on the thought, but to learn to simply redirect one's focus to the act of breathing. Children who are not able to comprehend the mindfulness aspect can be instructed simply to pay attention to counting to 5 during each inhalation and exhalation; they will derive similar benefits. Children can be told to use this deep breathing technique at times when they feel overwhelmed with physical or emotional stress, as long as they are not in a situation that requires their attention to something external (e.g., during an exam or if caught in a fire, attention needs to be focused on responding appropriately to these challenges).

Script for Focused Breathing (for Young Children)

"Remember how our bodies feel when we're stressed or thinking about things that remind us of the bad things that have happened? Our bodies get tense and tight, our hearts might start pounding, we're breathing real fast or maybe it's hard to catch our breath, and we might get headaches or stomach pains. We can reverse those feelings by practicing focused breathing. Deep, focused breathing is easy to learn, and we're going to do it now. The idea is to take slow, deep, controlled breaths, and to focus your attention on the breath going in and out. It helps if you breathe in a way we call 'belly breathing.' That means that your belly goes out as you take a breath in, and it goes in as you breathe out. One way to know if you're doing this right is to hold your hands over the lower part of your belly. [Demonstrate.] If you're lying down, you can put a little stuffed animal or book on your belly and check to make sure it is going up as you breathe in and down as you breathe out. Let's practice doing that a few times. [Practice.]

"Now we are going to add counting and what we call 'focusing' to the breathing. First, the counting: One way to do this is to take a deep, slow breath in, and as you exhale, say the number 'five' to yourself slowly, until all the air is out of your lungs. Then inhale slowly and deeply and say 'four' to yourself as you exhale. Keep going until you get to zero. Some kids find that it helps to do this belly breathing for several minutes, or even longer. If you decide to try that, you can count to five to yourself with every breath in, then count down to one as you exhale. If you keep breathing in this slow, controlled way, I think you'll notice that you feel more relaxed. Do you have any questions about how to do it? [Answer any questions.]

"The final part of this belly breathing is to focus your attention on the breath going in and out of your lungs. Imagine the air filling up your lungs all the way down to the bottom, and then all of that air coming out. As you pay attention to your breathing, you might notice that other thoughts come into your head [for younger children: 'You might notice your brain talking to you about other things.']. Don't worry if this happens; it's normal for that to happen. But what I want you to try when that happens is to return your focus to your breathing. Try not to be distracted by these other thoughts when they happen, just recognize them as thoughts that you have, and tell yourself that they can wait for later for you to pay attention to them.

"Are you ready for this? I'm going to do it, too. Let's try to close our eyes and start slow belly breathing. We'll try to do it for 3 minutes. If you stop in the middle or feel silly or self-conscious, that's OK, just start where you left off. I'll let you know when the 3 minutes are up. [Do belly breathing for 3 minutes.]

"How did that feel? Did you feel calm or relaxed while you were doing that? You can practice this at home during the week if you want to. It's a really nice way to fall asleep, and you can also do it when you're feeling worried, tense, or scared. Let me know how it works for you, OK?"

Script for Meditation (for Older Children)

"Remember how we practiced belly breathing and focused on the breaths we were taking? Was that relaxing for you? Now we're going to practice something very similar, which you have probably heard of before. It's called *meditation*, which is an ancient practice that Eastern religions have used for centuries. Studies have shown that, like belly breathing, meditation can reverse the effects of stress and trauma on our bodies, not just during the times that we are meditating, but all the time, if we keep practicing it. Do you have any ideas about what meditating is like? [The child may describe yoga or other impressions of meditation here.] Some people think about yoga positions that look really hard to do, or of people sitting on top of mountains in India. But the truth is, you can meditate anywhere. Meditation is simply the art of being totally in the present moment—aware of, but not wrapped up in, what is happening around you. One term for this is *mindfulness*. This term means that you focus on the present, and if your focus is interrupted by thoughts coming into your head, you observe your own thoughts but do not judge or act on them. This is a way to quiet our brains and our bodies, and to feel a sense of relaxation and peacefulness.

"I know this may sound funny at first, but if you pay attention, you will notice that your brain likes to be busy. If you just sit quietly, you will see that thoughts start coming into your head automatically. And we usually respond to these thoughts with other thoughts. Like if I think, 'I don't know what to do about dinner,' I might start thinking, 'Oh, I better go shopping. I don't think there's anything good to eat at home. I hope I'll have time to get to the store before I have to take the dog out for a walk . . .' on and on and on. Instead of doing that, in meditation, you would observe that thought, not judge it or feel like you have to do something about it, and then focus back on being in the moment. What you will find is that these random interrupting thoughts begin to happen less often and are less intrusive when they happen. This takes practice, though; it doesn't happen all at once.

"One way to keep focused on the present moment is to pick a phrase [in Eastern terms, a *mantra*] that makes you feel calm and peaceful and to repeat that to yourself as you focus on your breathing and on the here and now. Some kids pick a soothing word, such as *peace* or *love* or another one-syllable word. Other kids use a phrase from a song they like, or from a prayer. Is there any phrase that makes you feel peaceful and relaxed? [Help child come up with a mantra.]

"What we are going to do is practice mindful meditation here. Get into a comfortable position. [Child sits in a comfortable position.] Now close your eyes, and we are going to relax our bodies. I am going to talk calmly and very slowly as you focus on relaxing all the different parts of your body. I want you to relax your muscles, starting with your feet and moving up your legs. The feeling of relaxation is now moving up past your knees. Now relax your thighs and your butt. Now focus on relaxing your stomach and your back and chest. Focus now on relaxing your shoulders, your neck, your arms, your hands, and your fingers. Now relax your head. Now start belly breathing, and slowly as you exhale, say your special word or phase to yourself. Don't be concerned when other thoughts come into your mind. Just see that they are there and return calmly to your breathing and to your special word or phrase. Let's keep doing this for about 5 minutes. I will tell you when time is up, so don't worry about when to stop. [Practice meditation for 5 minutes.]

"OK, let's slowly finish, open our eyes, and sit quietly for a minute. How did that feel? Was that relaxing? I want you to try to practice this for at least 5–10 minutes every day, and tell me next week how it goes. I'm going to teach your mother how to do this, too, and you can also show her how to do it at home. I think you will find that your body will feel more relaxed, and when stressful thoughts or situations do come up, you will be able to cope with them more calmly as you practice this more."

PROGRESSIVE MUSCLE RELAXATION

Progressive muscle relaxation is another relaxation technique that can be particularly helpful for children who have difficulty falling asleep or who have many somatic symptoms. With younger children we use the analogy of a piece of spaghetti before it is cooked (stiff) versus after it is cooked (wiggly), or a tin soldier (stiff and tense) versus Raggedy Ann (loose and floppy). The therapist should explain that when our muscles are not relaxed, we feel tight and tense and sore, but when we relax those muscles, it helps us to feel easy and loose. Some children can relax their muscles simply by trying to "be like a piece of wet spaghetti" or "sit like Raggedy Ann." However, others will need specific instructions on how to progressively relax different muscle groups.

This technique is best practiced in a lying down position or in a relaxed sitting position; children may either lie down in the therapy room, sit in a comfortable chair, or practice at home. The child should be instructed to first tense (in order to accurately feel where these muscles are located) and then to relax one set of muscles at a time, starting with the toes, then the feet, then the ankles, etc., all the way up to the head, until every body part has been progressively relaxed. A typical script for directing children in progressive relaxation is offered in the following section.

Through practice, children can learn to fall asleep or relax specific aching body parts using this technique. However, even when nothing hurts and it is not bedtime, progressive relaxation may be helpful to children with PTSD symptoms, because the selective attention given to relaxing muscle groups typically precludes focusing on thoughts about the traumatic event at those particular times. In fact, instructing children to use these techniques when they have intrusive recollections of the trauma, such as at home or at school, may help them reverse the physiological symptoms of hyperarousal that typically accompany such thoughts, because tension and relaxation are incompatible.

The following script may be helpful for introducing children to progressive muscle relaxation techniques.

Script for Progressive Muscle Relaxation

"Let's review how your body responds to stress and trauma reminders. Your heart starts beating faster, your breath is faster and shallower, and your stomach and head might feel all tense and tight. What happens to your muscles during stress? [Child may answer, 'They get tight or tense, too.'] That's right, they tense up and get ready to respond to danger by fighting, fleeing, or freezing. Any of these responses require your muscles to tense, just like you were about to start a race in the Olympics. And that is not a feeling that is relaxing to most of us. So we want to reverse that tension in our muscles by purposely relaxing them. And by doing this, we can also reverse some of the other stress responses in our breathing and heart. So let's get started.

"We are going to relax our entire bodies, starting with our toes and working our way up to the tip of our heads, getting rid of every bit of tension as we go, until it comes out the top of our heads and floats away into space, leaving us relaxed and calm. This is a great way to fall asleep at night, and if you like, you can practice here in the office lying on the rug. Other kids feel more comfortable sitting in a comfortable chair. Where would you like to practice this in here? [Child picks a comfortable position.]

"Stretch out your body as much as is comfortable. Now I want you to focus your attention on the toes on your right foot. Are you focused there? I want you to tense up those toes as tight as you can, keeping every other part of your body relaxed. Can you do that? This is so that you can feel exactly where those toes are in your body. All right, now I want you to slowly relax them, until you can imagine them being as limp as a Raggedy Ann doll or a piece of wet spaghetti. Take a deep breath and imagine the oxygen going all the way to those toes as they relax completely. Okay, now I want you to focus on the rest of your right foot. Tense it up as tight as you can. Feel it? Now relax it slowly, keep relaxing it, until it feels totally limp and calm. Take a nice deep breath and feel the relaxation spread throughout your foot. Now focus on your right calf. Tense it up as much as you can. Now relax slowly until it's totally relaxed.

[Proceed to relax the right thigh and buttock, the left toes, foot, calf, thigh and buttock, right fingers, hand, arm, shoulder, left fingers, hand, arm, shoulder, lower back, moving up the spine to the upper shoulders, the neck, the scalp, the chin, mouth, cheeks, eyes, forehead, top of the head.]

"Now let the tension flow out of the top of your head and float away into space. Keep your eyes closed as you feel your whole body relax. If any part still feels tense, tense it up all the way now, then slowly relax it all the way until it is totally relaxed. Now take some deep belly breaths and keep breathing. [Continue breathing for 1–2 minutes.]

"How does your body feel now? How do your muscles feel? If this is relaxing to you, practice it at home and it will become even easier and work even better as your body becomes more used to relaxing itself. Try it some night to fall asleep and let me know how it works."

Other relaxation techniques, which involve movement of the entire body, may also be helpful for some children. For example, younger children may enjoy dancing the "Hokey Pokey," with the therapist using the "shake it all about" lines to demonstrate how to relax a specific body part. Therapists may encourage adolescents to bring in their favorite dance music and use dance as a relaxation method. Other therapists have found blowing bubbles (real or imaginary) to be helpful in inducing relaxation in children, who can then be directed to "float like a bubble."

Still other techniques can include helping children focus on one sense; for example, closing their eyes and letting a piece of candy melt in their mouth until it is all gone, then describing what it tasted like; listening to a tape of the ocean or a waterfall and describing what that sounded like; looking at a stained-glass panel of a rainbow or other colorful picture and describing that vision; or closing their eyes for 3 minutes and feeling a piece of velvet). These techniques help children maintain attention on the here-and-now. We encourage therapists to work creatively with each child to discover optimal ways of facilitating both mental and physical relaxation.

RELAXATION FOR CHILDREN WITH TRAUMATIC GRIEF

The relaxation techniques described above may be complicated for children whose trauma resulted in the death of a loved one, because so many of their previous positive memories or "safe places" may be associated with the deceased person, and thus these previously comforting memories or relaxing stimuli no longer feel safe or positive. Family rituals that used to represent security (e.g., snuggling with a beloved parent for a bedtime story) may now be trauma and loss reminders. These painful reminders may present a challenge to developing relaxation rituals, particularly at bedtime and especially for younger children who have lost a parent. The therapist will need to work closely with the parent and child to develop new comforting rituals that do not trigger trauma and loss reminders for either parent or child. Some families have repainted bedrooms, rearranged furniture, traded bedrooms, or in some extreme cases, moved to new homes, in order to not trigger such reminders. Developing new rituals for bedtime—new music, stories, games, songs, dance, massage and other relaxation techniques, may provide fun ways to bond together as a newly configured family.

RELAXATION FOR PARENTS

We include relaxation interventions for parents following exposure to traumatic events so that they can practice and reinforce these skills in their children and because they also typically need methods for managing their high personal levels of stress. In addition to the techniques described below, therapists may find additional helpful strategies for teaching stress management to parents in books such as *The Relaxation and Stress Reduction Workbook* (Davis, Eshelman, & McKay, 1988).

Focused breathing/mindfulness/meditation and progressive muscle relaxation techniques can be taught to the parent in the identical manner used with the child, as described above. Some parents may be interested in using focused breathing as a form of *meditation*, which is the practice of focusing one's attention uncritically on a single thing. Although the object of attention can be anything one chooses, it is often easiest to focus on one's own breathing. One reason why this practice is so helpful for reducing stress is that it is impossible to truly focus on more than one thing at a time; if the parent is able to focus on his/her breathing, he/she will not be able to focus on trauma-related thoughts or emotions (e.g., sadness, fear, anger) at that moment. Other benefits of meditation include learning that not all thoughts that come into one's head need to be attended to; that thoughts and feelings are not permanent but come and go frequently; and that most of the things we feel stress about are not happening right now but rather are related to the past or the future. These realizations can be very helpful when the parent is starting to feel overwhelmed in his/her attempts to deal with the traumatic event or with the challenges of daily living.

Although there are many methods and instructions for meditating, the easiest is the following:

"Find a comfortable position, begin deep breathing [as described above in the child section], and attempt to focus your attention only on your breathing. When other thoughts or feelings interrupt your focus, or your mind starts to drift to other things, bring your focus back to your breathing. Do this as many times as necessary and do not judge yourself for not being able to perfectly maintain your focus; this is normal. The benefits of meditation accrue from the effort of refocusing your attention, not from being perfect at maintaining it. Do this for 10 minutes a day to start, and try to work up to 15 or 20 minutes a day."

The therapist should encourage parents to spend 5 minutes in the session attempting this technique, because enhancing stress management in the parent may have a very positive impact on his/her availability to and support of the child.

OTHER RELAXATION TECHNIQUES

Parents and children may also benefit from any form of exercise that involves aerobic activity, because aerobic activity is known to decrease the physical manifestations of stress as well as to diminish symptoms of depression and anxiety. Parents should be encouraged to care for themselves by engaging in enjoyable, relaxing activities. Therapists may find it helpful to point out to parents that by participating in these activities, they are modeling the value of relaxation and self-care for their children. In addition, physical activities can be a great way for parents and children to achieve the physiological benefits of aerobic exercise while also enjoying opportunities to bond and spend quality time together.

TROUBLESHOOTING

What do you do if parents (or children) resist or refuse all attempts to develop personalized relaxation strategies?

Sometimes it is better to not insist in this situation. After all, "forcing someone to relax" is almost impossible. The therapist might say something like, "Relaxing is something that no one can force you to do. In fact, relaxing is the opposite of force, it is letting go of force and control. If a time comes when you change your mind and you want to learn to relax, I will be happy to help you. If you choose not to learn relaxation strategies, I will respect your choice, and I will try to understand the connection between that choice and some of the other symptoms you say [your mother says] you are having."

Some children are so traumatized that they do not know what pleasure feels like. How can you teach relaxation to these children?

Pointing out their fear of pleasure may be helpful to some children or parents. Pleasure may be associated with letting down one's guard, which may, in itself, be a trauma reminder for highly traumatized individuals. Sometimes simply saying, "Everyone has a right to feel pleasure. This is a safe place, you won't be harmed while you are here" may allow such clients to attempt relaxation exercises.

I see some teenagers who refuse to do any relaxation exercises. What do you suggest?

Let them bring in music and just listen to their music together. It is not necessary to do any physical relaxation exercises if they refuse to do these. It may be helpful to have crafts (knitting, crochet, embroidery, macramé) in your office that you can pick up and engage in while such clients are sitting listening to music. You can explain that these activities relax you and offer to show them how to do these activities. The idea would be to engage in 5–10 minutes of relaxing time during the session, however that might happen, to quiet the teen's and your mind.

What are some other ways to help children or parents get in touch with relaxation and pleasurable sensations?

Guided imagery may assist some children or parents in this regard. You can ask them to recall a time they felt peaceful and ask them to describe when that was, where they were, what it smelled like, what it looked like, etc., or have them describe an imaginary "safe place" and draw or imagine how this place might look, smell, sound, and feel.

Affective Expression and Modulation

As described earlier, children who have experienced significant trauma may have a predominance of painful, difficult feelings as well as dysregulation of affect. Many times these children are afraid that they will be overwhelmed by the strength of their feelings. Young children may not have the vocabulary to express the highly intense feelings they are experiencing. Affective expression and modulation skills help children express and manage their feelings more effectively. Moreover, by helping them gain a greater ability to express and modulate these frightening feelings, children may have less need to use avoidant strategies.

FEELING IDENTIFICATION WITH CHILDREN

Identifying their feelings is a relatively nonstressful way for children to begin talking about their feelings with the therapist. By sharing common everyday feelings with each other, the therapist is able to gauge the child's verbal and emotional ability to accurately identify and express a range of different feelings, while the child gets to know a little about the therapist, sees that the therapist has had "bad" as well as "good" feelings, and that the therapist is open about sharing these feelings with him/her. Thus, from the very beginning of treatment there is an attempt to establish and build trust and open communication between the child and therapist.

There are several different ways to help children enhance their feeling identification and expression skills. Some of these are described below. However, the therapist is encouraged to develop alternative ways of helping the child identify and talk about a range of different feelings. The therapist can initially ask the child to write down all the different feelings he/she can think of in 3 minutes (younger children may only be able to think of 5–10 feeling words, whereas adolescents will typically identify more feelings than they can write in 3 minutes). This exercise helps the therapist to estimate the child's adeptness at identifying different feelings. The therapist can then take turns with the child, picking feelings from the list and describing the last time each felt this particular feeling. Through the use of commercially available games such as Emotional Bingo (Mitlin, 1998), the Mad, Sad, Glad Game (1999), or the Stamp Game (for older children and teens; Black, 1984), the therapist can then have the child practice identifying feelings that occur in diverse situations (e.g., getting an "A" on a test, being teased at school) and identifying situations in which the child would experience a specific feeling (e.g., "Tell me a time when you felt embarrassed.").

Therapists can also make up their own feeling wheels or card games or engage children in making these during sessions as a fun activity during which a range of feelings can be expressed. Still another useful feeling identification intervention, particularly for younger children, is the Color Your Life technique (O'Connor, 1983). The therapist asks the child to pair different colors with specific feelings, and then to fill in different colors in different parts of a human figure to show where the child feels love, sadness, anger, etc. This technique facilitates the ability to access a variety of cognitions and feelings, and it is also fun for children because they are able to draw. In addition to appropriate identification and expression of thoughts and feelings, the therapist may find this technique helpful in identifying salient treatment foci. For example, an 8-year-old child's Color Your Life drawing included a large area of blue, which represented "feeling worried." When the therapist asked why the child felt "worried," the child said it was because other children at school teased her. In discussing this situation with the child's mother, it became clear to the therapist that only one child at school had teased the child on a few occasions. But due to this child's recent traumatic experiences, she had become overly sensitized to peer rejection. The information gained from the discussion with the mother was very helpful to the therapist and was a focus of treatment in the subsequent cognitive coping component of treatment for this child.

Older children may find the concept of "blended feelings" useful. Using different colors to represent "primary" feelings—that is, happy, sad, mad, scared—may assist children in identifying what components of these are present in other feelings. For example, if mad is red and scared is blue, a child might blend these feeling colors together (mad and scared, i.e., purple) to represent how he/she would feel if his/her mother was very late to pick him/her up after school. Some children might label this feeling *annoyed* whereas others might choose *edgy, uncertain,* or *impatient.* This activity helps children realize that (1) people often feel more than one feeling in a given situation, (2) these feelings might even seem opposite (e.g., feeling both happy and sad that you beat your brother in an important race), and (3) this is normal.

These games/activities should be continued until the child is able to accurately identify and comfortably discuss a variety of feelings in the appropriate situations. It should be noted that if feeling identification is introduced in an early treatment session, the therapist does not typically ask the child directly about feelings experienced during the traumatic event (although the child may spontaneously discuss this area, and if this occurs, the therapist should follow the child's lead). Because early treatment sessions are typically focused on building the child's comfort with, and trust in, the therapist, affective modulation sessions (like most sessions) should end on an upbeat, positive note, if possible (e.g., praising the child for doing well at feeling identification; allowing the child to choose a non-trauma-focused game to play for the last 5–10 minutes of the session).

AFFECTIVE EXPRESSION WITH PARENTS

Providing a comfortable atmosphere in which parents can share the full range of emotions they have experienced in the aftermath of the trauma(s) may help them to appreciate that the therapy session is a safe place where they can reveal even those less socially desirable feelings (e.g., being angry at the child for calling 911; feeling sadness or loving feelings toward the sex offender). Although it may not be appropriate to share some feelings with the child, it is important for the parent(s) to express and process the roller coaster of emotions that they may be experiencing. During the early sessions, in fact, it is most important to validate these feelings, acknowledging that there are no right or wrong feelings, just feelings that are more or less difficult to manage and endure. Indeed, learning about how parents are managing these difficult emotions often reveals clues about their coping strengths as well as weaknesses that can be utilized/addressed later in the course of treatment. A therapist who is advocating for the child might feel inclined to confront and/or correct a parent who is feeling angry at the child or expressing loving feelings for the individual who sexually abused the child, but doing so may not be appropriate early on, before the therapist has had an opportunity to develop a trusting therapeutic relationship. Nevertheless, the therapist *is* advocating for the child by encouraging the parent to utilize the sessions to work through feelings rather than expressing them directly or indirectly at home when children are present. Ultimately, therapy helps parents develop affective modulation skills and cognitive coping skills that not only help them manage their own emotions effectively, but also allow them to serve as more effective models of coping for their children.

When conducting parallel sessions with parents around affective expression and modulation, it is important to encourage them to look for and praise their children's efforts to express their emotions verbally. Helping parents practice reflective listening skills may be particularly valuable at this point because although parents usually can't change children's feelings, by actively listening they can reinforce children's efforts to share their feelings verbally as opposed to acting them out behaviorally (e.g., by fighting with siblings or peers). A homework assignment that encourages parents to note and acknowledge when their children express their feelings verbally will support in-session activities that require emotional expression skills (e.g., developing the trauma narrative). In session it may be useful to help a parent practice saying, "I understand that you're feeling mad because you can't sleep over at your cousin's house. I can't allow you to sleep over, but I'm glad you let me know how you're feeling." Making this type of limited, reflective statement is difficult for some parents because of tendencies toward debating, arguing, or attempting to fix the problem when children express negative emotions. Parents can be encouraged to see that responding in this way is an active response that helps children feel heard despite parental inability to fix the problem. It is particularly important for parents to accept that although they cannot undo the trauma that the child experienced, they can offer a great deal of support by participating in therapy and offering a listening ear when feelings and thoughts are expressed. For parents who are not yet emotionally prepared to respond to their child's questions and comments about the trauma itself, it can be very reassuring to know that simply reflecting back emotions that the child is sharing can be validating and helpful to him or her. In addition, parents can actively direct their children to share those feelings with their therapist as well.

THOUGHT INTERRUPTION AND POSITIVE IMAGERY

It may be useful to introduce thought interruption (or thought stopping) and positive imagery to some traumatized children early in treatment if they feel overwhelmed by trauma reminders (e.g., intrusive traumatic thoughts at bedtime or in school). However, this intervention may not be appropriate for very young children, who may find it confusing to be encouraged to talk and think about the trauma, on the one hand, and to stop thinking about it on the other. In general, we prefer that children not avoid trauma reminders but rather learn to master these. However, learning interruption techniques may be helpful as a *temporary* measure early in treatment before such mastery has been attained. Thought interruption is an affective modulation technique that can short-circuit the cycle of negative thinking that is often problematic for traumatized children (thoughts of the traumatic event lead to cognitive distortions, which lead to more upsetting thoughts and more cognitive distortions, and so on, or dwelling unproductively on very negative thoughts and scenarios). This technique can also prepare the child for cognitive-processing interventions because it teaches children that they *can have control over their thoughts.*

Thought interruption is a method of diverting the child's attention from the traumatic or otherwise upsetting thought and refocusing it on a nontraumatic replacement thought. In some ways, thought interruption is the opposite of what the child does when creating the trauma narrative (when we try to focus the child's attention on, rather than away from, the traumatic event itself). It may therefore seem contradictory to use both of these interventions in the same treatment model. However, some children benefit from encouragement to use thought interruption at times when they need to be focused on things going on around them, such as at school, when playing sports, or interacting with friends. Applying this technique teaches children, first and foremost, that they have control over their own thoughts—not just *which* thoughts they choose to focus on, but also *when* they focus on which thoughts. For children initially overwhelmed by intrusive reminders of the traumatic event, as well as distorted thoughts of their own responsibility or thoughts that exaggerate or catastrophize the reality of the situation (e.g., "I will never be happy again"), simply learning this principle can be very helpful.

Thought interruption is accomplished by putting a stop to an unwanted thought, either verbally (e.g., saying "Go away" or "Snap out of it" to the thought) or physically (e.g., wearing a rubber band around the wrist and snapping it to signal the desire to stop a thought). Some children may relate to the idea of "changing the channel" from a "show" that is focused on negative, upsetting stories to a more positive, enjoyable show. These children may prefer to "push the clicker" (press their finger on an imaginary channel clicker) instead of using a rubber band around their wrist. The next step is to replace that unwanted thought with a welcomed one ("Find a new channel to watch."). Some children prepare for thought interruption by having a positive thought or mental image ready—such as thinking about a special happy event, place, or experience (e.g., birthday, Christmas, amusement park). It may also be helpful for children to visualize a "perfect moment" (e.g., hitting a game-winning home run; being elected class president) to use for thought replacement. (This is the technique used in Lamaze childbirth.) This mental picture can be drawn and taken home as a prompt to use when applying thought stopping at home. Also, the more detailed description the child can give of this image (e.g., including sights, sounds, smells, tastes), the more this image can distract him/her from the intrusive thought.

Some therapists suggest that children visualize and draw a "safe place" to use during thought interruption as well as for general self-soothing. This may be either a real place where the child feels safe or an imaginary place. Some children ask to include the drawing of their safe place in the trauma narrative they create later in therapy, to assist them in tolerating trauma reminders during that portion of treatment. (We have found that doing so can be very helpful and encourage children to do this if they wish.) Teaching children thought interruption and positive imagery techniques helps to prepare them for the (likely) experience of ongoing reminders or negative intrusive thoughts about the traumatic event, both during the course of therapy and after therapy has ended. Mastering these techniques before creating the trauma narrative can help some children feel confident that if they start to feel overwhelmed while talking directly about the traumatic event, they will be able to interrupt or control these reactions.

POSITIVE SELF-TALK

Positive self-talk consists of focusing on the child's strengths instead of the negative aspects in any given situation. One could easily argue that there is nothing positive to be found about most traumatic events. However, many children have come through such traumatic events to find themselves stronger, more compassionate toward others, more thankful for their family members, etc. Children may benefit from recognizing (and focusing attention on) the fact that, despite great adversity, they are coping—and are often coping quite well. Positive self-talk requires the therapist to help the child recognize the ways in which he/she is coping well and to remind the child to verbalize these ways, particularly when feeling discouraged. Examples of positive self-statements are as follows:

> "I can get through this."
> "Things are hard now, but they will get better."
> "I still have a family, and they will help me."
> "Lots of people care about me and my family."
> "Some things have changed, but lots of things are the same as they were before this happened [example: I still do well in school, I still have friends, I'm still good at math]."

Although some children are naturally more optimistic in their outlook than others, optimism can be learned and practiced so that it becomes more a part of the child's life. Encouraging children to practice positive self-statements may enhance their ability to cope with adverse life events long after therapy has ended.

ENHANCING THE CHILD'S SENSE OF SAFETY

For many traumatized children, an important source of affective dysregulation is a real or perceived loss of safety. It is important to help the child express this feeling as well as to recognize the sources of support in the environment that can enhance the child's sense of safety *right now*. Before addressing safety issues with the child, the therapist should first ask the parent the nature and degree of social support available to the child at this time. Then the therapist can begin addressing safety issues with the child in a realistic manner, as demonstrated in the following:

> "Sometimes, when bad things happen around us or to people that we love, we start to worry that bad things are going to keep on happening. Sometimes it just seems like the world isn't a safe place. Have you been having any of these worries or feelings? [If the child responds affirmatively, continue.] When you are feeling this way, what can you do or say to yourself that might help you feel safe? Let's make a list. What do you count on to keep you safe? Who can

kids count on to keep them safe when their parents aren't around, like at school or when they are outside playing [typical answers: grandparents, teachers, police officers]? Who is keeping our country safe [typical answers: president, armed forces, FBI]?

If the child expresses clear misinformation or distortions regarding his/her safety, it may be helpful to point out all the people and social institutions that are working to keep the child safe now. For example, parents, teachers, police, child protection workers, judges, and the military may all be sources of protection (depending on the nature of the child's trauma; some of these may have contributed to the trauma, so it is critical to have knowledge about the child's actual situation). Helping the child come up with a clear and specific safety plan may also help achieve affective modulation, especially for children living under conditions of chronic and unpredictable threat (e.g., domestic or community violence).

The parent must be integrally involved in safety planning for the child. This phase can become complex, particularly in situations of domestic violence (e.g., the mother bringing the child to therapy returns to live with a violent partner, even though the child's safety plan stipulates that the child not be left alone with this partner). Unrealistic safety plans will not help children feel safer, and they may undermine children's trust in the parent and therapist. In these situations it is better for the therapist to acknowledge that, unfortunately, there may be no guarantee of safety in the child's situation but that they (i.e., the therapist and child) can plan ways to maximize the child's ability to minimize risk and harm and to respond optimally to danger. If appropriate, the therapist should also attempt to access other community resources, if these are available, to protect the child and family (e.g., through child protection, police, alternative housing, victim advocacy, witness protection, and other programs).

Practicing specific personal safety skills to enhance a child's responses to dangerous situations that might occur in the future can be very helpful. However, when possible, it is best to postpone the active practicing of these skills until later in therapy, after the child has completed much of the trauma narrative. This postponement is important because the narrative is intended to reflect the child's actual experience and response at the time, not what the child thinks he/she should have done. A great deal of focus early in treatment on personal safety skills may inadvertently encourage inappropriate feelings of responsibility and/or guilt for not having done what the therapist is now suggesting.

(Personal safety skills training is reviewed in greater detail in the final trauma-focused component.)

ENHANCING PROBLEM-SOLVING AND SOCIAL SKILLS

Children who have experienced chronic or interpersonal traumatic experiences may have learned maladaptive coping responses in social situations (e.g., attempting to bully their way through any social encounter). Initial assessment and/or ongoing observations as well as parental and child reports may reveal difficulties with respect to managing peer relationships and social interactions. Some children's repertoire for dealing with socially or otherwise challenging situations may be very limited. Specifically, such children may have only one or two responses to ambiguous or difficult situations (e.g., extreme anger or withdrawal). Novel situations or peer problems are common triggers for affective dysregulation in these children. Enhancing problem-solving and social skills may assist these children in affective modulation. Many of these skills involve aspects of cognitive processing, *in vivo* exposure, and other TF-CBT components, but because they are provided in this model primarily as a method of affective modulation, they are described in this component.

Problem solving involves several steps that can be summarized as follows:

1. Describe the problem.
2. Identify possible solutions.
3. Consider the likely outcomes of each solution.
4. Pick the solution most likely to achieve the desired outcome and implement that choice.
5. Evaluate your choice to see how it worked.
6. If it didn't work out as hoped, try to figure out what went wrong.
7. Include what you just learned the next time a problem arises.

Here is an example: Joseph has experienced many years of family violence. He has witnessed his father beating his mother, and he has been physically abused by his father and older brother. Joseph is fearful at home and tries to avoid his father and brother as much as possible. At school Joseph is perceived as mean, unfriendly, and isolated. He is also having trouble with angry outbursts. For example, when other children accidentally bump into him on the playground or in the classroom, he "explodes," immediately hitting them and screaming "Get away from me!" As a result, other children do not like him and are starting to ostracize him. This is causing Joseph to feel even worse about himself. He says, "My father and brother don't like me, and now kids at school hate me too."

Joseph is experiencing PTSD symptoms in response to chronic trauma. Unexpected physical contact serves as a trauma cue for him; he interprets any such contact as traumatic and responds to it with avoidant behaviors at home and aggressive reactions at school. His peers and teachers do not understand the source of his behaviors and see him as mean and scary. He does not see the connection between his own trauma symptoms, his subsequent behaviors toward peers, and how these behaviors affect his peer relationships.

Although helping Joseph gain mastery over trauma cues will be an important part of his treatment, it may be possible to teach him some problem-solving and social skills earlier in treatment to alleviate some of his peer problems and help him with affective modulation in the meantime. Consider the following dialogue between Joseph and his therapist:

THERAPIST: Joseph, it sounds like you're having some problems with kids at school because they don't understand how you feel, and you are having trouble making them understand. Like when they bump into you or intrude on your physical space that really upsets you, and they don't get that, right?

JOSEPH: Yeah, it really bothers me when people get in my face.

THERAPIST: So let's go through what usually happens when someone "gets in your face." What happens next?

JOSEPH: I yell at him, or I push him away or maybe I hit him if he doesn't back off.

THERAPIST: And your mom mentioned that you've gotten detention for that a few times too, right?

JOSEPH: Yeah.

THERAPIST: So here's the problem: You don't like when people get in your face. Right?

JOSEPH: Right.

THERAPIST: OK, let's write this down (gets Problem-Solving Worksheet to fill in [see Figure 4.1 on p. 99]). The problem is that you don't like people to get in your face. Now, let's think about all the possible things you might do when that happens. We already know a few things you have tried, right?

JOSEPH: Huh?

THERAPIST: You just told me what you've tried so far, what you usually do when kids get in your face.

JOSEPH: I tell them to back off.

THERAPIST: I think you said you yell at them. Is that the same as telling them or asking them to back off?

JOSEPH: Yeah, basically.

THERAPIST: You know what, I think maybe there is a difference, at least maybe to the kid on the receiving end of that. For me, it feels a little different if someone says politely "Would you please back off" versus yelling "GET OUT OF MY FACE, YOU JERK!" Does it feel different to you?

JOSEPH: (*Laughs.*) Yeah, I guess.

THERAPIST: So we have two different possible responses right there. One is to yell something rude, the other is to calmly ask the person to back off. And I think you mentioned a few other options you've tried. . . .

JOSEPH: You mean, hitting the guy?

THERAPIST: Exactly. So let's fill in all of these options under possible response. Can you think of any others?

JOSEPH: Not really.

THERAPIST: How about just walking away?

JOSEPH: Sure, if I want to get beat up.

THERAPIST: Are you sure that's what would happen? Have you tried that before?

JOSEPH: No, not really.

THERAPIST: Let's just add it to the list for the heck of it, OK?

JOSEPH: OK.

THERAPIST: OK, so now let's try to imagine what would happen if you tried each one of these reactions. Some of them you already know the answer to, because you've tried them several times, right?

JOSEPH: I guess so.

THERAPIST: So let's fill those in.

JOSEPH: OK. With the hitting, I know I'll get sent to the principal's office.

THERAPIST: And what will the effect be on your relationship with the kid you hit?

JOSEPH: He won't like me.

THERAPIST: Is that the outcome you want?

JOSEPH: I don't know.

THERAPIST: Oh, I'm sorry, maybe I'm confused. I thought you said you wanted more kids to like you in school. Do you want this boy to dislike you?

JOSEPH: No, I want him to like me. I just don't want him in my face.

THERAPIST: OK, so there are two bad outcomes to hitting him: You get in trouble with the teacher and principal, and the kid you want as a friend ends up not liking you. How about yelling at him?

JOSEPH: It's pretty much the same thing. And other kids get into it too sometimes, like they stick up for him and call me names, so that doesn't work out too well either.

THERAPIST: OK, so now we have two other possibilities. What do you think would happen if you told him in a firm but low voice not to bump into you or not to get in your face? Or maybe even to give you some space? How about like this: "Hey, listen, I need some space right now, OK?" How do you think he would take that?

JOSEPH: I don't know. It might be OK. He might laugh at me.

THERAPIST: I guess there's no way to know unless you try it. Are you willing to give it a try the next time something like this happens?

JOSEPH: Yeah, I can try it.

THERAPIST: There's another part to this situation that might be a problem. Do you think the next time this kind of situation comes up you could stop, take a breath before reacting, and then say something like this before you yell or hit? Or do you think hitting or yelling is so automatic that you won't be able to help yourself? Because if it's really a split-second reaction, there are other things you can learn and practice for that.

Possible responses	Possible outcomes	Good or bad outcome?
1. Ask to please back off.	1. ?	1. ?
2. Yell at him.	2. Get in trouble; he doesn't like me.	2. Bad outcome.
3. Hit him.	3. Get in detention; he really doesn't like me; other kids also don't like me.	3. Really bad outcome.
4. Just walk away.	4. ?	4. ?

FIGURE 4.1. Problem-solving worksheet for affective expression and modulation.

JOSEPH: No, I think I can try it.

THERAPIST: OK, and we are going to come back to this list after you try it and fill in what happens. If it doesn't work out, we are going to go to this other possibility of walking away and think about that one some more. Finally, in this next week, I want you to take this home and see if you can come up with any other possible responses. Then if you get a chance, try them out this week, and see how they work, and next time we will look at how they work out too. OK?

JOSEPH: OK.

SOCIAL SKILLS BUILDING

Social skills encompass a variety of abilities and behaviors, some of which are relatively easy to teach (e.g., taking turns, listening to others, acceding to the wishes of others at times), others of which are more complex and difficult (e.g., accurately reading social cues, understanding illogical and unjust peer hierarchies of popularity). If available, providing social skills group treatment is an ideal approach for enhancing children's development of these skills, particularly for traumatized children, who can benefit greatly from meeting peers who have also experienced traumatic events. Group work can be a very powerful intervention for removing stigma related to trauma; that is, children get to meet children whom they like and admire and who have also been traumatized, and if those children are OK, in the child's perception, the child's self-image may also improve.

In the event that such groups are not a possibility, individual therapy can also provide some social skills building. Teaching the basics of the skill to be learned (e.g., taking turns), modeling it for the child (with the therapist taking the role of another child), and then practicing with the child in therapy sessions can help the child acquire social skills that then can be practiced in real-life situations. The therapist should check back with the child to see how the skill practice has fared in subsequent weeks and offer strategies for corrective action if the child's attempts were less than successful. Older children can role-play with the therapist difficult peer interactions they are experiencing and, together, troubleshoot a variety of alternative strategies for addressing difficult peer situations. Sometimes these practice sessions can help children recognize that there are times when peers are mean for no reason, and no matter what strategies are tried, they can't become friends with everyone. In addition, by reenacting these situations in role plays, the therapist has an opportunity to praise the child for demonstrating effective, assertive communication skills, while also offering constructive feedback that will enhance his/her responses. It is often helpful for the therapist to coach the child on verbal as well as nonverbal assertive responses, such as making appropriate eye contact and demonstrating confident body posture.

Parents should also be involved in reinforcing children's social skills by practicing with them at home. In addition, parents can be helpful in selecting appropriate candidates for the child to invite for play dates, arranging activities with the peer's parents, providing transportation, troubleshooting with the child if problems arise during these interactions, and providing praise and reassurance between sessions for the child's attempts at appropriate social interactions.

MANAGING DIFFICULT AFFECTIVE STATES

The goal of learning the above skills is for children to be able to better manage difficult affective states. In essence, they are developing a number of "tools" to select from their "tool kit" for when they become distressed. Several additional skills are required to successfully modulate difficult affective states. First, children need to be able to recognize when they are starting to feel distressed and intervene to modulate these feelings before they become overwhelmed. Next, children need to select an affective modulation skill (or combination of skills) to use that is appropriate to the situation at hand. Children might be encouraged to generate a list of several different ways they can soothe themselves. A sample list is included in Appendix 1 in the Affective Modulation Handout. From the possible range of self-soothing activities, the child needs to find a way to "match" the best activity to the particular circumstances. For example, positive self-talk or thought interruption might be the best skill to use when feeling stress while taking a test at school; positive imagery or seeking parental support might be the best skill to use for intrusive trauma reminders at bedtime; problem solving might be the best approach for dealing with anger at peers; and so on. The therapist should work with the child to examine specific situations in which he/she is having difficulty with affective regulation and develop individualized plans for how to use these or other affective modulation skills to address these difficulties. At each subsequent session, the therapist should "check in" with the child to see how these strategies have worked. If they have not been successful, additional skills may need to be added or other adjustments to the plan will need to be made. Parents should be enlisted to reinforce the child's attempts at affective modulation when appropriate, as discussed below.

AFFECTIVE MODULATION FOR CHILDREN WITH TRAUMATIC GRIEF

Children who lose loved ones due to intentional acts such as homicide, terrorism, or war are likely to need help with particular emotions. The fact that someone intentionally set out to injure or kill a child's loved one may lead to intense feelings of anger, fear, hatred, or wanting to get even (revenge). It is important that the therapist assure the child that many children have these feelings and that the feelings are OK because they are not actions and therefore not harmful by themselves. Rescue fantasies (described on p. 128) can be much more intense for children whose loved ones died as a result of traumatic events; their survivors' guilt may also be more strongly felt and more difficult to resolve.

Thought interruption techniques may need to be adjusted for children who have experienced a traumatic death. These children should not replace traumatic thoughts with thoughts of the deceased loved one while he/she was still alive. Such thoughts, although initially comforting, can easily segue into upsetting reminders of how the loved one died. It is more helpful to guide the child to focus on a more neutral scene wherein the deceased person is not present.

Enhancing the child's sense of safety may be very difficult after someone has died, particularly when the death was intentional. Providing *realistic, age-appropriate* reassurance is important. Parents as well as therapists should provide such information. The therapist should also explore with the child what would help the child feel safe *right now*. In addition to the interventions suggested on pp. 158–165, the therapist might also include a discussion of the family's "backup" plan for keeping the child safe. The therapist should use clinical judgment as to whether raising this issue will worsen the child's fears or bring into the open a concern that lingers beneath the surface for many children who have already lost one parent.

If the child has no backup safety net—for example, if the child lives in a foster home and has no contact with biological relatives—it is especially important to discuss with the child what might help him/her feel safer. Developing an ongoing relationship with a Big Sister, Big Brother, or mentor in the community may enhance such a child's sense of safety and belonging. All children need to feel that, if their current caretaker were to die or become unable to care for them, there is a plan in place that provides for their future well-being. Discussing such a plan with traumatically bereaved children is very helpful in enhancing their sense of safety. In many cases optimal development of this plan is achieved jointly among the therapist, child, and parent so that the parent can assure the child that the plan will actually be put into place, if necessary, in the future. Although making such a plan may seem morbid to those of us who have not been in this situation, it can be very soothing to a child who is fearful and affectively dysregulated due to ongoing heightened anxiety following the death of one parent.

AFFECTIVE MODULATION FOR PARENTS

Thought Interruption and Positive Distraction

All of the techniques described above may be useful for parents as well as their children. In addition to the techniques described in the child treatment section, therapists may want to suggest (if the above strategies are not successful) the use of *paradoxical intention* for affective modulation in parents who are troubled with intrusive thoughts about the traumatic event their child experienced (Frankl, 1985). This technique can involve requiring the parent to think about the upsetting thought for a predetermined period of time, after which he/she must use thought interruption to stop thinking about it. The paradox is that trying one's hardest to think about something makes it easier to stop thinking about it. For example, take the parent who fixates on worries about the child before going to bed at night. The therapist could instruct the parent to worry about those matters in the morning only, not at night. At night she must use thought stopping to interrupt those thoughts and replace them with "perfect moment" thoughts or other positive images. Each morning the parent might set a timer for 3 minutes, during which time she is *supposed* to think about nothing but these worries, as intensely as she can for those 3 minutes. When the timer goes off, she should stop thinking about those worries for the rest of the day. Some parents report that their mind wandered during the 3 minutes, and that such focused worry was difficult to sustain all at once (probably for the same reason that it is hard to stay focused on one's breathing without distraction). Other parents report that giving themselves "permission" to worry lessened their need to do so. Typically, paradoxical intention should only be used if cognitive-processing techniques have been unsuccessful in reframing inaccurate or unhelpful thoughts.

Like their children, parents should be encouraged to identify relaxing activities (e.g., exercising, reading, talking to friends, listening to music, taking a bubble bath) that help them modulate and self-soothe upsetting affective states. Therapists can help parents give themselves permission to relax and enjoy a few stress-free moments each day, even though their child has gone through a horrible experience. Therapists may want to point out to parents that by doing this they model positive coping for their children and help them believe that they can still enjoy happy moments, and deserve to do so, even in the midst of dealing with a life trauma. It is also helpful to point out to parents that being stressed, hyperalert, or vigilant at all times is not going to help their children recover any more quickly or protect them from future harm. To the contrary, children are most likely to adjust well after trauma when their parents are able to cope effectively, communicate openly, and begin to enjoy life again. For these reasons it is critical to encourage the development of practical and effective coping skills in parents.

Positive Self-Talk

This technique can be used to challenge pessimistic thoughts that either arose following the traumatic event or that the parent held previously but which have become stronger since the trauma or loss. Such pessimistic thoughts may include the following:"

"I can only be happy if my child is happy."
"I can't trust anyone anymore."

"Being strong means I should never feel upset/unhappy/angry."
"Good parents always know the right thing to say to their children."
"It's horrible when things go wrong in life."
"Some problems have to be avoided because they are just too hard to handle."

Positive self-statements to challenge these might include the following:

"I can find things to be happy about, and this will set a good example for my child."
"Most people are good at heart, and many are trustworthy."
"Being strong means doing what you have to do, and I am doing that."
"I am a good parent; I do lots of good things for my child, including bringing [him\her] to therapy, even though it is painful."
"Things going wrong is just a part of life; facing challenges can make you stronger."
"I am facing the hardest thing that has ever happened to me, and that takes a lot of courage."

The therapist can encourage and reinforce these positive self-statements by telling the parent true observations the therapist has made about him/her. For example, the therapist might tell the parent that he/she (the therapist) admires the parent's strength in the face of adversity; that the parent is doing a great job of keeping a positive attitude and modeling this for her child, etc. Hearing this type of genuine comment from the therapist may have a very significant impact on how the parent views him/herself and/or his/her child. It is also helpful early in treatment to offer statements that will inspire hope and confidence in the treatment approach, such as reminding the parent that the treatment has much scientific support of its efficacy in helping children and parents overcome posttraumatic emotional difficulties.

TROUBLESHOOTING

How can I tell if anger is related to trauma or to externalizing behavioral problems?

Making this distinction is a difficult clinical dilemma. Sometimes the timing of symptoms may help make this determination. For example, knowing that a child's anger management problems clearly preceded the onset of trauma exposure may clarify that anger is a problem independent of trauma. However, even if trauma did not precipitate the onset of anger management problems, any current aggressive behaviors must be addressed directly, regardless of their origin. Specifically, hurting other people or damaging property is unacceptable for any reason, and the child must accept responsibility for his/her actions and choices. The problem-solving and anger management skills described earlier may be helpful in this regard. Other interventions described in abuse-focused cognitive-behavioral therapy (Kolko & Swenson, 2002) may also be appropriate for such children.

How do you manage children who are so emotionally "blocked" that they can't express any feelings at all?

Almost all children can express some feelings; some are unable to differentiate between feelings (e.g., they will always say they feel "mad" regardless of the situation) and others will seem very emotionally blunted if they are, in fact, depressed. Such children may need to participate in many more sessions devoted to affective expression or modulation skills in order to enhance trust in the therapist, engage them in the therapeutic process, or overcome other barriers to open affective expression. Therapists may explore with parents the source of children's extreme reluctance to share feelings in such situations; parents may be able to share valuable insights in this regard. For example, if a child was severely punished by a battering parent for expressing negative emotions in the past, the therapist can use this knowledge to assure the child that this will not happen in therapy, where expression of all feelings is welcome. This child's mother could also be a powerful influence on the child in therapy if she were able to encourage the child to express feelings in the therapy session. Sometimes children enjoy competing with their parents to see who can come up with the longest list of feeling words. The therapist might then consider a nonthreatening joint child–parent activity as part of an early feeling identification session for such a child in order to encourage affective expression. For example, parent and child might engage in a fun "feeling charades game" in which a non-trauma-related feeling is demonstrated nonverbally and the other party has to guess the feeling.

What if a teen says he/she cannot describe any feelings?

Ask him/her to list feelings that other teens might have. It may be easier to start talking about feelings in the third person and gradually move to more personalized feeling expression. The therapist can assist in this process by taking turns: "OK, you describe a time when one of your friends might have felt anger. Then I'll tell you about a time when I felt angry." If the therapist does not force the issue, the teen will probably start opening up about his/her own feelings within a few sessions.

What if a child or teen is really affectively dysregulated? Is it safe to proceed to the next components of treatment?

For *severely* dysregulated children, it is probably important to master some affective regulation skills before proceeding further in treatment. One of the core skills might be identifying triggers to upsetting emotions and ways to better manage these triggers. Parents can also be enlisted to help children in this regard. Until some reasonable degree of affective stability is achieved, and cognitive processing is mastered, it is probably not a good idea to proceed to the trauma narrative. However, many children will continue to have some degree of anxiety, sadness, and anger related to the trauma even after they have completed the trauma narrative. Thus the operative word here is *severely* affectively dysregulated children; it is expected that all children receiving this treatment will have a moderate degree of affective dysregulation.

Cognitive Coping and Processing I
The Cognitive Triangle

Efforts to make sense of traumatic experiences are often reflected in children's and caregivers' thoughts. The term *cognitive coping* refers to a variety of interventions that encourage children and caregivers to explore their thoughts in order to ultimately challenge and correct cognitions that are either inaccurate or unhelpful (Beck, 1995; Seligman, Reivich, Jaycox, & Gillham, 1995). Knowledge and life experiences help individuals make sense of traumatic events. However, given children's limited experiential and knowledge base, they may be particularly prone to inaccurate or dysfunctional thoughts about traumatic experiences, and these thoughts can negatively influence their developing views and belief system.

The first step in helping children and caregivers utilize cognitive coping skills involves the recognition and sharing of internal dialogues. These internal dialogues, however, can be difficult to capture and share, especially when they are ingrained, repetitive, and/or include stigmatizing thoughts. Thus it is best to begin the discussion of cognitive coping with simple non-trauma-related exercises. For example, encouraging children to share the first thing they said to themselves before getting out of bed in the morning and before speaking out loud may help them understand what is meant by thoughts of internal dialogues (e.g., "I'm tired"; "I don't want to go to school"; "I wonder what I can have for breakfast"). Some children may not even be aware that all people talk to themselves. It can be a welcome relief to young children that they are not the only ones who have ongoing conversations with themselves.

Many children and parents do not realize that they can choose to change their own thoughts, and that doing so can change their feelings and behaviors. This idea is the basis of the "cognitive triangle," depicted in Figure 5.1.

Educating children and caregivers about the connections among thoughts, feelings, and behaviors is an essential element of psychoeducation about cognitive processing. The first step in this process is to practice feeling identification, which is described in Trauma-Focused Component 4 (pp. 87–89).

The next step in explaining the cognitive triangle is to help the child and caregiver *recognize the distinction and relationship between feelings and thoughts.* This psychoeducation may have already occurred during feeling identification exercises if the child mistakenly identified a thought instead of a feeling (e.g., when asked, "How would you feel if a girl in your class never talks to you?" the child answered, "I would feel like she hated me."). If this misunderstanding occurs during feeling identification activities, the therapist should point out to the child that he/she just shared a thought, or idea, rather than a feeling, and again ask the child what he/she would be feeling in that situation (e.g., sad, angry, rejected, unloved). Younger children may understand "thoughts" as "our brains talking to us."

In order to teach the child how to distinguish between thoughts and feelings, the therapist might explain the following:

"Most people assume that feelings come from inside of us, of their own accord, and we have no control over what feelings we have or when we feel them. However, this isn't really accurate. Most of the time, we have feelings in response to the thoughts we had at that

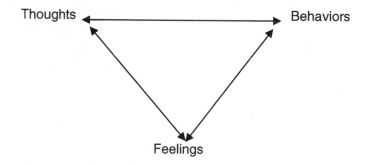

FIGURE 5.1. The cognitive triangle.

time. Sometimes we get used to having certain thoughts so often that we aren't even aware that we are experiencing them. These are called 'automatic thoughts' because we have them without conscious awareness, out of habit, and just assume that everyone else would have the same thoughts as we do. But we often have thoughts that are inaccurate, or not helpful, and these thoughts lead to feelings that hurt us rather than help us. Let me give you some examples."

The therapist then can give examples such as the following (these should be tailored to each individual child's interests, age, and gender, so that the child is easily able to relate to them):

"Say there's a girl in your class, and she never talks to you. When you walk by her, she looks down or looks the other way. If your thought in this situation is, 'That girl hates me,' you might then feel sad or angry. But let's suppose that, instead of thinking 'She hates me,' your thought is, 'Gee, she must be really shy.' How would that make you feel?"

The therapist allows the child to answer. Typical responses might be, "I wouldn't feel so sad," "I would feel sorry for her," etc. Once the child understands this concept, the therapist should present a series of scenarios in which the child has to *identify both a thought and a feeling that results from that thought*. If the child names a feeling first, the therapist should ask, "What thought did you have that made you have that feeling?" or "What were you saying to yourself when you were feeling that way?" Sample scenarios and appropriate responses include the following:

1. Your mother blames you for something your little brother did.
   Thought: "She's not being fair."
   Feeling: hurt, mad.

2. Your teacher announces that there will be a pop quiz today.
   Thought: "Math isn't my best subject. I'm gonna get an F."
   Feeling: scared, worried, mad at teacher.

3. You get invited to a dance by a boy you really like, who you thought didn't like you.
   Thought: "He does like me!"
   Feeling: excited, happy.

The next step is to encourage the child to learn how to *generate alternative thoughts that are more accurate, or more helpful,* in order to feel differently. Some children may understand this concept better if the therapist compares it to changing the channel on the TV: "If you don't like what you are seeing on one channel, you can switch to another channel to find a better show. Finding a more accurate or helpful thought may similarly involve some 'channel surfing' until you find a thought that feels better." Some young children may find the use of "thought bubbles" beneficial. The therapist draws cartoon characters with bubbles above their heads, representing the characters' thoughts. Children are encouraged to "fill in the bubbles" by answering the question "What is this person's brain telling [him/her]?" If the child identifies an inaccurate or unhelpful thought, the therapist might say, "Can't we come up with something else for this child to say to [him/herself] that might help [him/her] feel better?" This technique is comfortable for many children because it uses characters similar to the cartoon and comic book characters with which they are familiar. Other children might like the analogy of putting on different colored sunglasses: "The situation you see is the same but you see it 'in a different light.' " For example:

1. Your mother blames you for something your little brother did.
   More accurate thought: "Mom won't be mad at me once she knows the truth."
   New feeling: hopeful.

2. Your teacher announces that there will be a pop quiz today.
   More helpful thought: "I've done all my homework, I should do OK."
   New feeling: calm, reassured.

3. You get invited to a dance by a boy you really like, who you thought didn't like you.
   More accurate/helpful thought: "I don't need to change the first thought I had—it was accurate, helpful, and made me feel good!"

The final step in explaining the cognitive triangle is to help the child recognize the relationship among thoughts, feelings, and behaviors, as well as the relationship between our behaviors and how other people act in response to us. (This is the same approach used in teaching children problem-solving skills and may promote healthier coping in children with PTSD or other trauma-related problems as well.) Younger children may be better able to understand this process through reading a story that illustrates the use of cognitive reframing. A good example is *The Hyena Who Lost Her Laugh: A Story about Changing Your Negative Thinking* (Lamb-Shapiro, 2000). The relationship among thoughts, feelings, behaviors, and results (i.e., how other people respond) can be demonstrated by using the above examples or others that are more applicable to an individual child, as the following:

> Your mother blames you for something your little brother did.
> *Scenario A:* "Mom's not being fair."
> > *Feeling:* mad
> > *Behavior:* You say "I hate you!" and run to your room.
> > *Result:* Mom punishes you.
>
> *Scenario B:* "Mom won't be mad once she knows the truth."
> > *Feeling:* hopeful
> > *Behavior:* You calmly explain to your mother that you didn't do it.
> > *Result:* Mom apologizes for blaming you unfairly.

The therapist should practice this exercise with the child by discussing several different scenarios in which the child can *change his/her feelings and behaviors by thinking differently.* If possible, these scenarios should be from the child's real life. However, unless the child spontaneously gives as an example his/her thoughts and feelings related to the traumatic event, exploration and revision of these cognitions should be done in conjunction with creating the child's trauma narrative (i.e., once the child's trauma-related cognitions have been identified through creating the trauma narrative). Often children are told repeatedly that the traumatic event was not their fault, that they should try to stop thinking about it, etc. Children are sensitive to these adult expectations, and particularly after a frightening experience, are often anxious to please caring adults. This desire to please may lead to a reticence to discuss their true thoughts, especially their most horrifying or "unacceptable" thoughts. Thus, when asked in therapy about trauma-related thoughts prior to creating the trauma narrative, children may minimize or avoid revealing these cognitions. Once children have mastered discussing the traumatic event by creating the trauma narrative, therapists are more likely to hear their true cognitions in this regard.

Because cognitive processing of the child's trauma typically occurs after creation of the trauma narrative, we have included this part of the cognitive-processing component after Trauma-Focused Component 6.

TYPES OF INACCURATE AND UNHELPFUL THOUGHTS

The many types of inaccurate and unhelpful thoughts that children have fall into typical patterns that have been described in various ways. For example, research has demonstrated that people who attribute negative events to *personal* (internal), *pervasive* (global), and *permanent* (always) causes are more likely to become depressed than people who attribute these events to external, specific, and transient causes (Seligman, 1998). Let's use as an example two children who both fail the same test. The first child says to himself, "I failed that test because I am stupid, I can't learn anything, I will never be any good at anything." This statement is *personal* (attributes the failure to his own shortcomings), *pervasive* (assumes that he is stupid at everything, not just at learning what was on this particular test), and *permanent* (assumes that it is unchangeable in the future). The second child says to herself, "That was a really hard test. I thought I knew that chapter, but I guess I have to study harder to learn it all. I will study harder next time and do better." This statement, although attributing some personal responsibility to the child for not studying the right material, makes neither pervasive nor permanent declarations. The second child is not only less likely to feel badly about herself for failing but is also more likely to study harder for the next test.

Children may more easily learn to recognize maladaptive thinking patterns when they are described in the following styles (Mueser, Jankowski, Rosenberg, Rosenberg, & Hamblen, 2004):

YES OR NO YASMINE

Yasmine sees everything as either *yes* or *no*; either the glass is all full or all empty—there is nothing in between. For example, if she doesn't get an A+ on the test, she might as well get an F.

> "If the world isn't perfectly safe all the time, it is always dangerous."
> "If you can't trust every man [woman], you can't trust any man [woman]"

OVER-AND-OVER OLIVER

Oliver sees the world as a neverending pattern of one bad thing happening after another, just because one bad thing happened to him once. He always jumps to conclusions that bad things are going to happen, even before they happen. Sometimes this makes bad things more likely to happen! For example, Oliver might think:

"If my friend doesn't want to talk to me after school today, then that means he will never want to be my friend again."
"I was in a car accident once, so I will be in a car accident again."

CALAMITY JANE

Jane always focuses on the worst possible outcome in every situation. No matter what happens, she starts to think "what if?" thoughts, leading to thoughts about the worst-case scenario. For example, if she gets a bad grade on one test, she thinks, "This means I will fail the whole year. That means I will never get into a good college, and I will be a total failure. My life might as well be over right now."

"If I have nightmares about the shooting, it means I am going crazy. They will put me in the hospital and I will never get out."
"My father is late picking me up . . . something bad might have happened to him like it did to my brother . . . he might even have gotten shot just like my brother . . . oh my God, I bet he's dead!"

NO-WAY NORA

Nora is always thinking negatively: No matter what's going on, she always finds something to be down about or finds some way to think things won't work out well. This attitude keeps her from seeing the bright side of things, even when things are going well, and pretty much guarantees that she will feel miserable a lot of the time. For example, if Nora gets invited to a party, she thinks, "Probably no one will talk to me anyway, and I'll have an awful time. There's no use in me even going, because I'll have such a terrible time."

"Nothing's ever going to work out for me, so why even bother?"
"Domestic violence has ruined me for nice boys, so I might as well be with bad ones."

In this early stage of therapy, the most important message for children is the importance of becoming aware of their thoughts as well as the potential influence of those thoughts on their feelings and behaviors. Children should also be encouraged to share internal dialogues in the course of therapy, particularly when they begin to develop their trauma narratives. In fact, as children become more comfortable talking and writing about their traumatic experiences, they are likely to reveal dysfunctional and/or inaccurate thoughts that may underlie their emotional difficulties.

THE COGNITIVE TRIANGLE FOR PARENTS

The therapist should introduce the cognitive triangle to the parent in a similar manner that was used for the child, or using an example such as the following:

"Suppose you go to a movie and you see two women you know only slightly. They look your way from across the lobby but continue to talk to each other without coming over to say hello to you. Let's take a look at what your thoughts might be and how those thoughts might affect your feelings and behavior. Say your thought is 'They are gossiping about me.' How would that make you feel? [Parent answers 'embarrassed,' 'angry,' 'hurt.'] If you felt embarrassed, what would you do? What would your behavior be in this situation? [Parent answers 'walk away,' 'glare at them,' 'leave the theater.'] Now what if, instead of thinking they are gossiping about you, your thought is, 'They must not have seen me.' How would you feel then? [Parent answers, 'neutral,' 'curious about what they are discussing.'] Now if you felt nothing or were curious, what might your behavior be? [Parent answers, 'I might go over and say hello to them'; 'I would just go in and see the show.'] So, you see, the objective reality of what happened in those two scenarios was exactly the same, but changing the thought made a big difference in your feelings and behavior in that situation."

The therapist can then ask the parent to identify a situation in which he/she was feeling bad and have the parent identify the thoughts that led to those bad feelings. The parent should then be asked to generate alternative thoughts that might lead to less distress. As is the case with the child, it is not necessary for the therapist to examine parental cognitions about the child's trauma at this point, unless the parent spontaneously raises this topic. Early in treatment the goal is to introduce the cognitive triangle and encourage parents to identify inaccurate or unhelpful thoughts occurring in their daily lives and to learn how to feel better by examining and reframing these.

Cognitive coping can be used to challenge pessimistic thoughts that either arose following the traumatic event(s) or were held previously but have become stronger as a result of the trauma or loss. Such pessimistic thoughts may include the following:

"I can only be happy if I am in a romantic relationship."
"There is only one true love for everyone and I lost [him/her]."
"Being strong means I should never feel [upset/unhappy/angry]."
"Good parents always know the right thing to say to their children."
"It's horrible when things go wrong in life."
"Some problems have to be avoided because they are just too hard to handle."

Coping statements to challenge these might include the following:

"Lots of things make me happy; I will try to do one fun thing for myself each day."
"It's too soon for me to think about loving someone else, but someday it may be possible."
"Everyone feels upset sometimes, and this does not mean I am not strong."
"No parent always says the right thing all the time. I am doing the best I can do."
"Even though I have gone through something horrible, my child and I are still here."
"This is really hard, but so far I am still handling it OK without running away."

As noted previously, the therapist can encourage and reinforce these cognitive coping statements by telling the parent true observations the therapist has made about the parent's courage in the face of huge obstacles and adversities.

ENHANCING THE SURVIVING PARENT'S SENSE
OF SAFETY

In situations of traumatic parental death in a family, children often exhibit increased feelings of fear, vulnerability, and mistrust; the surviving parent also often feels fearful, unsafe, and distrustful. It is important for the parent to communicate a general sense of safety to the child and to provide an environment of emotional support. In order to enable the parent to do this, the therapist needs to optimize the parent's own sense of safety. The therapist might begin by asking whether the parent has been experiencing a decreased sense of safety and a sense that the world will never feel safe again. If the parent answers affirmatively, the therapist might say something like the following:

> "I hear you saying that it feels like you will never be able to move on since the terrorist attacks, but I wonder how the people living in Northern Ireland or Israel manage to carry on amidst the constant fighting and terrorist attacks. Clearly, many people are choosing to stay there. There must be something positive that keeps them there. If we asked them, I wonder what they would say. What do you think they would say? [Allow the parent to answer. If the parent does not respond, the therapist may suggest the following.]
>
> "I have heard some people in these situations say things like 'This is my home, my country, and I will not let these few evil people chase me away or frighten me into not living a full life.' Others have said, 'Our way of [life/religious freedom, etc.] is worth fighting for and even worth dying to preserve. We have to give a message to terrorists—that they cannot take away our freedom or way of life—by standing up to them even when we are afraid.' "

What might we learn from people who are living in situations that seem very unsafe from an objective viewpoint? What can they teach us about finding inner safety in our lives?

TROUBLESHOOTING

How do you handle situations in which a child's culture has myths or beliefs that are inaccurate or unhelpful with regard to trauma (e.g., those that partially blame a girl for being the victim of rape, for not being a virgin)?

This is a difficult topic. To our knowledge, there are no cultures that truly hold such beliefs, yet every culture has some small minority that claims that its culture or religion does hold these beliefs. So the problem is clarifying and highlighting the true values of their culture or religion. We have found the best way to do this is to go to the "source"—that is, go to religious or cultural leaders for assistance in these situations, as we are rarely in a position ourselves to say what different cultures or religions stand for. In this regard, a church elder or other respected community leader can affirm for the family and child that their culture does not blame the victim for rape, etc. This approach has been more effective than trying to convince a child that we know more about his/her culture than he/she does when we clearly do not. Going to the source is also helpful to the family members who may feel shame and now are better able to provide support to the child.

What do you do if a child cannot come up with alternative (more accurate or helpful) thoughts?

The therapist can help the child by offering alternative thoughts and discussing each with the child. Or the therapist might ask the child for help with another child he/she is seeing in therapy; for example: "I am seeing another boy [girl] in treatment and I could really use your help. He [she] keeps thinking that no one wants to be his [her] friend. What else could he [she] think in this situation? Do you have any ideas about what I could say to him [her]? I really think you're the guy [gal] to help me out here.").

How can you help parents who are so preoccupied with the legal system that they cannot refocus their thoughts on how to be helpful to their child?

This is a situation in which cognitive processing can really be helpful if parents will use it to their benefit. Usually there are aspects of the legal system beyond the parent's immediate control, whether related to the trial of a sexual abuse perpetrator, a custody hearing of an abusive intimate partner, the homicide trial of the murderer of a child's parent, etc. Regardless of the parent's degree of anger and desire for revenge, there is probably nothing he/she can do to change the legal situation. Holding to the thought "I can't be OK until the legal proceeding is resolved" will likely interfere with the parent's well-being and parenting. The therapist can assist the parent here by pointing out that this thought may not be helpful or optimal and that a more hopeful thought may be "I can find a way to be OK while I'm waiting for this to be resolved; I can focus on caring for myself and my child." Furthermore, as a therapist, you can behaviorally reinforce this message by explaining that you would like to focus your individual time with the parent on the steps that he/she can take to help support his/her child, rather than spending too much time discussing the legal proceedings, because this is less likely to influence his/her child's well-being.

Parents can be encouraged to begin tracking their trauma-related thoughts at home from very early in treatment. It can be helpful to record thoughts on forms such as the type provided in Appendix 1 in the Practicing the Cognitive Triangle during the Week Handout. However, even when the parent has not recorded his/her thoughts in writing, completing this type of homework in session is helpful; ask the parent to identify a time during the week he/she was thinking about the trauma and feeling particularly distressed. Helping a parent capture the thoughts that were streaming through his/her mind at the time is a critical step in identifying and disputing inaccurate or unhelpful thoughts.

TRAUMA-FOCUSED COMPONENT 6

Trauma Narrative

Creation of a trauma narrative (also referred to as *gradual exposure* or GE) has been utilized in the treatment of children who have experienced sexual abuse (Deblinger & Heflin, 1996; Cohen & Mannarino, 1993) and children exposed to community violence (Pynoos & Nader, 1988), disasters (Goenjian et al., 1997), and single-episode traumatic events (March et al., 1998). One of the goals of creating the trauma narrative is to unpair thoughts, reminders, or discussions of the traumatic event from overwhelming negative emotions such as terror, horror, extreme helplessness, shame, or rage. Over the course of several sessions, the child is encouraged to describe more and more details of what happened before, during, and after the traumatic event(s), as well as his/her thoughts and feelings during these times. When done correctly, the therapist encourages the child, in carefully calibrated increments, to talk and write about increasingly upsetting aspects of the traumatic event, so that each step is only slightly more difficult than the preceding one. This calibration is not always easy to accomplish, because the therapist may not know what aspect of the event was most difficult for the child, and only learns this when the child gets to that part in the narrative. The therapist can encourage the child to "put yourself back there in your mind" and remember all the details "just like it was happening now." Many children will not be able to tolerate doing this until they have spent one or more sessions describing these events, thoughts, and feelings from their present perspective.

Deblinger et al. (1990) originally conceptualized the creation of the trauma narrative as an exposure procedure whereby repeated reading, writing, and elaboration of what happened during the trauma desensitized the child to trauma reminders. Hence, physical and psychological hyperarousal upon exposure to such reminders was decreased. This improvement would then decrease the child's need to avoid such reminders, thereby decreasing PTSD symptoms and allowing the child to resume more normal functioning. In addition, when describing the traumatic experience(s), the child was encouraged to share his/her thoughts and feelings so that the therapist could begin to identify and ultimately correct dysfunctional thoughts and developing beliefs that might underlie ongoing emotional and behavioral difficulties.

Work with traumatized adults conducted by Pennebaker (1993) and Pennebaker and Francis (1996) also suggested that creating only a trauma narrative was not sufficient to improve psychological or physical health, but that it *was* essential to integrate thoughts and feelings about the traumatic events into a consistent and meaningful experience. Other research with adults experiencing recent trauma suggests that adequate coping capacity, stress management and cognitive processing skills, and a focus on one's place in the trauma and in the present are also necessary in order for the creation of a trauma narrative to be beneficial rather than deleterious (Gidron, Peri, Connolly, & Shalev, 1996; Klein & Janoff-Bulman, 1996; Foa, Molnar, & Cashman, 1995). Thus, our current conceptualization of the trauma narrative is that in addition to desensitizing the child to traumatic reminders and decreasing avoidance and hyperarousal, this process also enables the child to integrate the traumatic experience into the totality of his/her life. In this way, the trauma is only *one* part of the child's life experience and self-concept, rather than being the defining aspect of both. This distinction involves metacognitive abilities; that is, the abilities to think about and evaluate one's own thoughts and experiences. We have found that even younger children have some ability to engage in metacognitive processing. In practice, creating the trauma narrative and cognitively processing the trauma experience co-occur, to some degree, and these components must occur interactively in order for the child to successfully integrate the trauma experience and its meaning into a larger optimal self-concept.

Prior to initiating the sessions in which the child creates the trauma narrative, the therapist should introduce him/her (and the parent, as discussed below) to the theoretical basis of this intervention. Children and parents may be understandably concerned about directly discussing the specific events surrounding the trauma; PTSD-based avoidance may play a factor in this reticence, or it may simply be due to the discomfort that is commonly experienced in discussing upsetting events. We have described the reason for creating the child's trauma narrative as follows

(Deblinger & Heflin, 1996), which the therapist may modify to fit the needs of the individual child:

"It is very hard to talk about painful things, and often children and parents try to avoid doing this. In fact, they say things like 'let sleeping dogs lie,' and wonder if it is a good thing to bring back memories of sad things. We tell kids and parents that if they had been able to put those memories behind them, the children would not be having any problems, and they would not be coming here to therapy in the first place. It's like when you fall off a bicycle and skin your knee on the sidewalk, and all that dirt and all those germs get into the wound. You have two choices about what to do with that wound. You can ignore it—not wash it off or put any medicine on it—and hope that it gets better all by itself. Sometimes that works fine. But other times, if you do that, the wound will get infected. Infections don't usually get better by ignoring them; they get worse and worse. Your other choice is to wash the wound carefully, getting all the dirt and germs out of there. That stings, it hurts at first, but then the pain goes away, and it doesn't get infected and can heal quickly. In the end, it hurts a lot less to clean out a wound than to let it get infected. Creating the trauma narrative, or telling the story of what happened, is like cleaning out the wound. It might be a little painful at first, but it hurts less and less as we go on, and then the wound can heal. Just like when you clean out a wound, if you rub too hard or too fast, it will hurt a lot more than if you go more carefully. We try to go at just the right pace in telling your story so that it never hurts more than a little bit. You can let us know at any point if we are going too fast for you, and we will slow down."

Once the child understands the rationale for creating the trauma narrative (i.e., talking about the upsetting aspects of the traumatic event a little bit at a time so that it is less and less painful/frightening/overwhelming over time), the therapist can help him/her begin to tell the trauma story. This process is most typically accomplished by having the child create a book that tells the story about the traumatic event(s). However, the therapist can begin this process by having the child write a chapter about him/herself and a favorite activity recently enjoyed. As noted previously, this step allows the child to practice creating/writing a narrative about a positive experience, which is likely to enhance his/her skill in writing a trauma-related narrative.

Still, despite this practice, some children write very little, perhaps just one sentence, the first time they attempt to write about the trauma(s). For example, one child wrote "My father cut my mother in the face." In such situations, the therapist can ask the child to verbally describe what he/she was doing at the time this incident occurred, and to describe what happened next, and after that, and so on. Once the child has verbally described these events, the therapist suggests that the child now write down what he/she just described. Although it is also essential to encourage the child to describe and write down the thoughts and feelings he/she experienced during the traumatic event(s), it may sometimes be more productive to have the child first describe his/her perception of the facts, and to return to the beginning and ask about thoughts and feelings only after these have been written. Interrupting the child in the flow of his/her narrative may make it harder for him/her to keep focused on the event and may also encourage avoidance of describing further details of what occurred. Many children enjoy having the therapist act as the "secretary" who writes as the child dictates the narrative.

Because most children are reticent at first to talk about their own traumatic experience, we usually introduce the trauma narrative component by reading a book such as *Please Tell* (Jessie, 1991; for sexual abuse), *A Place for Starr* (Schor, 2002; for exposure to domestic violence), *All Kinds of Separation* (Cunningham, 1992; for parental separation due to child abuse, parental substance abuse, or hospitalization), fill-in-the-blank books in the Creative Healing Book Series (Alexander, 1993a–1993d), *A Terrible Thing Happened* (Holmes, 2000; for exposure to crime or violence), *Molly's Mother Died* (Holmes, 1999a), *Sam's Dad Died* (Holmes, 1999b), *The Brightest Star* (Hemery, 1998), *Goodbye Mousie* (Harris, 2001) (for exposure to traumatic death), *Bart Speaks Out* (Goldman, 1998) (suicide), or *Brave Bart* (Sheppard, 1996) (unspecified trauma). These books make it possible for the child to read about another child's experience with similar traumatic events, and they create a structured format for the child to write about his/her own experience. Once the therapist has read such a book to the child (or the child and therapist have taken turns reading it out loud), the therapist should suggest that the child can write his/her own book about what happened to him/her. Almost all children will agree to this suggestion when they receive the appropriate encouragement and support. The therapist may act as a secretary and do most of the writing and reading for children who have not yet learned to read or for children who prefer not to do the writing and reading themselves because of reading disabilities or avoidance.

It is often helpful to suggest that the children start with non-traumatic information; for example, telling something about themselves, what they like to do, with whom they live, where they go to school, etc. Then they can be encouraged to describe the context leading up to the beginning of the traumatic experience (e.g., their relationship to the perpetrator prior to the beginning of the interpersonal violence or the traumatic death; the day before the disaster, accident, or violence occurred). Finally, children are encouraged to move to the details of the traumatic experience(s) itself (themselves).

Writing the entire descriptive narrative of what happened may take several treatment sessions, depending on how difficult it is for the child to recall, describe, and write these details, how much detail the child recalls and is willing to provide, and how long a time period is covered in the child's description. After the child has completed each segment of writing (whether in one session or over the course of numerous sessions), it is helpful to ask the child to read what he/she has written thus far; the child thereby gains mastery in verbalizing the details of the trauma and is readier (i.e., refocused) to write the next segment of the description. If the child is reticent to read what he/she has written, the therapist may read it out loud to the child thereby exposing the child to a retelling of the traumatic event. Over several repetitions, the child typically experiences progressively less extreme emotional reactions and physiological reactivity. If the child continues to experience a high degree of reactivity, relaxation techniques can be utilized during the session (as described in Trauma-Focused Component 3).

In some situations the child may not know all of the exact details about the traumatic event. For example, a child might have gotten out of a burning house or lost consciousness after a car accident or shooting and not know what other people in the house/car experienced prior to their severe injuries or deaths. This absence of information may lead the child to imagine horrifying scenes of loved ones suffering. In such a case, it is important for the child to verbalize and write these imagined traumatic reminders in the book. Methods for neutralizing the intense negative emotions that accompany these traumatic reminders are discussed below.

Once the child has completed his/her description of what happened during the trauma, the therapist should ask the child to read it from the beginning and include thoughts and feelings he/she was having during the events described in the narrative. It is not unusual for the child to also recall additional narrative details during this part of the process, and he/she should be encouraged to add these at the appropriate parts of the book. Initially, the goal is to help the child simply describe all of his/her recalled thoughts and feelings; exploring and challenging these should be put off until they have been recorded in the book.

At some point in the writing of this book, the therapist should ask the child to describe the worst moment, worst memory, and/or worst part of the traumatic event, and include this in the book. The therapist, for example, might ask the child to include in the book the aspect of the trauma that he/she never thought he/she would tell anyone. The child should be encouraged to describe this aspect in as much detail as possible, including drawing a picture of the memory. While doing this, many children reexperience some degree of fear, revulsion, sadness, or anger. The therapist should encourage the child to write these feelings and describe the physical sensations that accompany them (i.e., tight stomach, rapid breathing). However, if the child seems overwhelmed by these feelings, it is helpful to remind him/her that these are only feelings, and that they are related to something that happened in the past, not something that is occurring in the present. The use of puppets to describe these events may be helpful with younger children to provide initial distance between the description and possibly overwhelming feelings (Worden, 1996). The therapist or the child should describe in the book what the child enacts with the puppets, and in subsequent readings the child should be encouraged to discuss these events, thoughts, and feelings more directly. Relaxation techniques may be helpful at these junctures, and the child can be reminded that he/she has control over his/her thoughts. Children may also benefit from a brief distraction task (e.g., talking for 5 minutes or less about something unrelated to the traumatic event, such as what they did at school that day) at these points. In our experience, children are typically able to describe the "worst moment" without overwhelming, negative emotions, provided they have spent adequate time earlier in the session (or in previous sessions) gradually describing and gaining mastery over less horrifying aspects of the traumatic event.

Once the child has written the full narrative of his/her memories, thoughts, and feelings about what happened, cognitive-processing techniques are employed to explore and correct cognitive distortions and errors, as described in the following section. At the end of each session that is focused on the child's writing of the trauma narrative, the therapist should be sure to praise the child for his/her efforts and to give a developmentally appropriate reward, such as a material reinforcer (e.g., stickers) or a brief enjoyable activity (e.g., playing a game unrelated to the traumatic event).

Some therapists use the Subjective Units of Distress Scale (SUDS) to help children quantify their degree of distress within each session. This scale uses fear thermometers or children's faces depicting varying degrees of distress. If the child's SUDS progressively decrease during sessions in which the trauma narrative is created, this progress can be pointed out to him/her as a sign of how well the child is handling this challenging task.

Therapists should also encourage children to include at the end of the trauma narrative ways in which they are different now from when the traumatic event(s) happened and when therapy began; what they have learned or how they have grown from going through the traumatic event(s) and creating the trauma narrative, and advice they might give to other children who have experienced similar types of trauma. This intervention assists children in thinking about how the trauma experience fits into the totality of their lives and helps them integrate both positive and negative effects of this experience into their concept of themselves, the world, and their relationships with others. Children may elect to add or modify parts of the trauma narrative during the cognitive-processing component of treatment (described below); they should be encouraged to incorporate any new cognitions and metacognitions into the trauma narrative.

We have often been asked how to structure trauma narratives for children who have experienced more than one type of trauma or for children whose entire lives have been characterized by trauma. In these cases we suggest that the child guide the therapist as to which traumatic experiences to include in the book and in what order. For example, one child had experienced both sexual abuse and domestic violence; the worst episode of domestic violence in this girl's view occurred after she disclosed the sexual abuse, when her mother confronted the sexual abuser. This man threw the mother down the steps, where she lay bleeding and unconscious. The child's trauma narrative started before the sexual abuse, described the events that occurred during the multiple episodes of abuse, and then described the domestic violence, including the above episode. After rereading this narrative, the child then decided to add several episodes of domestic violence to the beginning of the narrative, because these had preceded the sexual abuse. In this manner, creating the trauma narrative seemed to help this child contextualize both the sexual abuse and the domestic violence.

For children who have had multiple foster placements and/or multiple traumatic events, we have sometimes suggested that they create a "life narrative" rather than a trauma narrative. Some children have enjoyed making a "timeline" of their life like those made in history class; others have preferred to put together a picture album starting with their birth, describing why they left each placement and what events (both traumatic and pleasant) occurred in each home, up until the present time. We have found that this timeline helps children to recognize that, even when multiple traumas have occurred, their lives have also had some fun, happy events. It also allows us to point out to them how strong they must be to have gotten through so many difficult and challenging times. For children who prefer to create a story on the computer, the Storybook Weaver computer program may be useful. Here are a few examples of children's trauma narratives.

Trauma Narrative 1: 12-Year-Old Latino Girl with Traumatic Grief

How My Mother Died

By Isabella

Chapter One: This is about me.
My name is Isabella. I am 12 years old. I go to school #4. My hobbies are acting and painting. The people in my family are my dad, my sister, and dog. I like chocolate the best.

Chapter Two: My mom.
My mom was smart. She read a lot. She took me to the library. She really loved books. When I was little, she read to me all of the time.

Chapter Three: Mom died.
My mom died on a really warm day. She was coming home from work and she was shot. She was shot by a stranger. When she died, I was at my best friend Rosie's house. Dad came to Rosie's house and told me the news. I couldn't stop crying. Rosie hugged me. Dad hugged me hard. He was crying, too. I was mad that I didn't get to say goodbye to my mom. The police don't know who killed my mom.

Chapter Four: The rest of the story.
On the night my mother died, my aunt and uncle came over. They were sad, too, but they made me feel better. They told me how much my mom loved me and that my mom knew how much I loved her. At the funeral home, all of my family and friends came. It seemed a little bit like a party, but then I would think "I won't see my mom anymore," and then I felt sad again. Why do people do terrible things like killing other people? Why do people die when you need them? My mom won't be able to go to the library with me anymore. When it was time to leave the funeral home, that was the worst part. I would never see my mom again. I felt really mad. Back at our house, I talked with my dad. Thank goodness I still have him.

What I've learned:

1. Talk to someone who cares about your feelings.
2. I survived something really hard.
3. I'm glad I came for counseling.
4. It is OK to talk about my mom.

Trauma Narrative 2: 9-Year-Old White Boy,
Witness to Domestic Violence

Hi, my name is Michael. I live with my mother and two sisters, Erica and Emily. We used to live in Heywood. Now we live in Plymouth Hills. We moved because of what happened at my house. We used to live with my dad. He did bad things. I miss my dad. One day he and my mom had a big fight. My father and mother were screaming. My father was hitting my mother. I was hiding in my room. I was really scared and shaking. I tried to not hear, but it was too loud. I hid under the covers, but they was too loud. Then my sisters came and the police found me under the covers. They took my mom to the hospital and my dad went to jail. I didn't want my dad to go to jail, so I felt sad. We went to my neighbor's house until my mom got out of the hospital. Then we went to live in Plymouth Hills.

My dad and mom have had many fights before this. Now I know that they can't live together because they don't know how to get along without fighting. My dad kept hurting my mom. He has to learn not to hurt anyone just 'cause he runs everything in our house. My mom tells me that she will not let him come back and live with us. I love my mom and my dad. The End.

It is important to note that narratives vary greatly in length and detail. Very young children may offer relatively few words but powerful drawings, whereas teenagers often create narratives that are detailed, lengthy, and incorporate events that occurred before and after the traumatic experience(s) themselves.

TRAUMA NARRATIVE FOR CHILDREN WITH TRAUMATIC GRIEF

In war, disaster, and terrorist situations, children lose loved ones but may not know under what circumstances; bodies of the deceased are sometimes not recovered and children are left to imagine the last moments of their loved ones' lives. These tragic circumstances may lead the child to imagine horrifying scenes of suffering prior to death. Moreover, when the death of a loved one occurs as a result of acts of terrorism, homicide, or the like, children may experience a variety of thoughts and feelings related to the intentionality behind the act. As noted previously, feelings of anger, helplessness, and/or thoughts of revenge are not uncommon and, indeed, are to be expected. However, when these thoughts and feelings become intrusive and repetitive—that is, become trauma reminders—they should be addressed and resolved through direct discussion. In such a case, it is important for the child to verbalize and write these imagined traumatic reminders in his/her trauma narrative. Methods for neutralizing the intense negative emotions that accompany these traumatic reminders include the following intervention.

It is important for the therapist to encourage the child to talk about any thoughts and feelings that may be related to the intentionality of the death. During the trauma narrative component it may be helpful to encourage the child to explicitly describe these thoughts and feelings in the narrative. These may include rescue fantasies as well as revenge fantasies. The therapist may want to use a prompt, such as: "If you had special powers and could have made things turn out differently, what would you have said or done to change what happened?" The child should be encouraged to include these thoughts in the narrative as well. The therapist can then point out to the child that these thoughts are normal and indicate how much the child wishes the events had not happened the way they did. The therapist should then assist the child in recognizing that no one can change the past because the past is over. However, we all have the ability to change some things in the present and the future by our own actions. Most of all, we can change our own thoughts, feelings, and behaviors, as discussed with the child during the cognitive-processing component (Trauma-Focused Component 5). The therapist should ask the child what he/she could do *right now* to make things "come out better" in the present or future. The therapist should then encourage the child to think about specific ways to achieve symbolic corrective action in the present and future. These can be included in the child's trauma narrative or in a special meaningful activity the child engages in outside of therapy (e.g., joining Students against Drunk Driving if their loved one was killed by a drunk driver).

Older children can sometimes achieve resolution by engaging in some benevolent or symbolic activity that gives them a sense of power and closure. They may choose to volunteer to help others (e.g., work in food kitchens for the homeless) or become more involved in religious or community activities that "do good" for others. The therapist can encourage youngsters to think along these lines: "We can't change what happened, but we can sometimes do things that are good in response to the bad things other people have done. Sometimes that can help us begin to feel better, too. Can you think of something that could make you or others feel better right now?"

Finally, the therapist should encourage the child to write a corrective story that can be placed at the end of the trauma narrative. The therapist may prompt the child to include a page entitled "I Would Like the Story to Turn out Like This in the Future" or "What I Look Forward to in the Future," or "My Happy Ending." For example, some children hope to grow up to become a rescue worker or to work for world peace or religious tolerance as ways to prevent such terrible events from happening again.

Although some therapists believe that acting out aggressive rescue or revenge fantasies (e.g., flying to the top of the World Trade Center and carrying victims to safety, or killing the terrorists before they crashed the plane) leads to resolution of underlying feelings, we have found that, in many cases, aggressive reenactment may serve as "practice" to become a victimizer (Ryan, 1989). We therefore believe that aggressive behaviors should be addressed behaviorally outside of therapy, and although verbal expression of aggressive urges is acceptable in treatment sessions, the therapist should actively intervene to resolve these. For example, the therapist can point out to the child that such actions reflect what he/she *wishes* could have happened, and then help the child move toward more constructive thoughts/fantasies/actions through which to make the world safer in the future.

SHARING THE TRAUMA NARRATIVE
WITH THE PARENT

The therapist should start by directly explaining the rationale for creating the child's trauma narrative, using similar analogies (cleaning out the wound) to that used with the child. The parent may wish to discuss concerns about this procedure, and the therapist should encourage such discussion. It may be helpful to predict that the child may not initially enjoy this part of therapy, may resist attending therapy once creation of the trauma narrative begins, and may even show more (transient) symptoms during this phase of treatment (see also p. 62 in "Trauma-Focused Component 1"). The therapist should ask the parent to tell him/her if this happens, so that therapy can be adjusted to the child's comfort level. It is our experience that almost all children can tolerate creating the trauma narrative if it is correctly calibrated and they are given the appropriate support from the therapist and parent. The parent should be reassured in this regard and also told that the child will not start creating the trauma narrative until he/she has gained some stress management skills as well as some comfort with the therapist and the therapeutic process. It may also be helpful to share with the parent that in our centers, at the conclusion of treatment, the majority of families have told us that creating the book or talking about what happened to them was the most helpful part of treatment.

Finally, the therapist should explain that in addition to resolving the child's PTSD symptoms, another goal of creating the trauma narrative is to allow the child to become more comfortable in discussing his/her thoughts and feelings with the parent, even when they are upsetting. The therapist should explain that this is important because the parent should be the person to whom the child can come with any problems or worries, whether about the traumatic experience or anything else. Showing the child, through joint sessions, that the parent is able to tolerate discussing even the most upsetting subjects (i.e., the trauma) and that the parent responds to the child in a supportive and helpful manner will encourage the child to talk to the parent about any problems that arise in the future. Most parents are eager to accomplish this goal and support the creation of the child's trauma narrative when it is explained in this manner.

Once the child embarks on creating the trauma narrative, it is usually helpful to share with the parent the narrative the child is writing or creating. With all children, but especially with adolescents, it is important to acknowledge that some aspects of the narrative may be shared with parents. It may also help the adolescent to know that the therapist will also be sharing some of what the parent is discussing with him/her. The therapist can still remind the youngster that something that is not dangerous to the adolescent or others can be kept confidential if he/she doesn't want it to be shared with his/her parent(s). Some children may object to sharing the narrative on the grounds that they do not want to upset the parent with reminders of the traumatic event. It is important for the child to learn that the parent can tolerate discussing the trauma. If the child is still concerned about this issue, the therapist should reassure him/her that the parent is discussing similar things in his/her own sessions and wants to share the child's experiences, thoughts, and feelings. The therapist can offer the reassurance that, if the parent starts to get overly upset, the therapist will stop reading the narrative; at the same time, the therapist reassures the child that the parent will be able to handle reading his/her book.

In other cases, the child may be afraid that the parent will be mad about things he or she has written (e.g., if the child expressed anger at the parent or if the child believes the parent did something to cause the traumatic event). In this case the child should be reassured that the parent wants to understand what the child is going through and that the therapist does not believe the parent will be upset or angry at any of the child's thoughts or feelings. The therapist must then be prepared to address the child's concerns with the parent and to resolve these issues so that the parent can remain supportive of the child and therapy.

To prepare the parent for hearing and seeing the child's trauma narrative, the therapist should ask the parent to describe his/her own experience of the trauma. The therapist can begin by asking how the parent heard about what happened—where was the parent, who told him/her the news, what was his/her first reaction, etc. Having the parent talk through the sequence of events and his/her thoughts and feelings may be very difficult, and adequate time should be available during the session to allow the parent to complete this narrative without interruption. It is important that the parent also have adequate time to regain his/her composure before the end of this session, because it is not helpful for the parent to return to the waiting room in tears (many children will believe that such parental distress is related in some manner to things the children did or said in therapy).

The parent should then be reminded that the child is also describing this experience in therapy, in the form of a book, which the therapist will share with the parent as it is being written. If the child has already started the trauma narrative, the therapist may then share it with the parent. It is important for the therapist to praise the child's ability to the parent and to praise the parent for encouraging the child to attend therapy and share memories, thoughts, and feelings about the trauma, even though it is painful.

As the child continues to create the trauma narrative in subsequent sessions, the parallel parent session should be devoted largely to the parent's reading of the child's book and discussion of his/her reactions. As with the child, at each subsequent trauma narrative session the therapist should reread the book out loud to the parent. This repetition provides ongoing exposure of the parent to the child's traumatic experience, with the goals of improving the parent's ability to tolerate hearing the child's description of the event and helping the parent process and integrate what happened to the child in an optimal manner. In this context, it is important to assess the parent's emotional reactions and to elicit the thoughts that may underlie his/her very strong emotional responses.

Again, helping parents identify and dispute dysfunctional thoughts (e.g., "This is all my fault—I should have protected my child better") and supporting them in utilizing effective coping strategies will enhance their ability to emotionally support their child. The culmination of the trauma narrative component is the conjoint child–parent sessions, which are described in Trauma-Focused Component 9.

Some parents may try to "correct" the child's book (e.g., noting that the child described events out of sequence or had some other detail wrong). The therapist should explain that unless these details are directly relevant to the child's functioning or otherwise having a clearly negative impact, the parent should not "correct" the book when meeting jointly with the child or talking with the child about it. Occasionally the child has inaccurately heard, remembered, or interpreted details related to the traumatic event, subsequent investigation, legal proceedings, etc. In this regard, an informational question–answer period (i.e., the parent says, in essence, "You can ask me anything") in a joint session may be necessary to clarify these questions. This type of intervention is particularly helpful for children who are unsure of the accuracy of their own information and clarification from a joint session will ultimately affect the outcome of their trauma narrative. The point is not to describe the exact objective reality of the trauma, but to help the child describe, and gain mastery over, his/her most upsetting, intrusive memories and images of the trauma. It is also beneficial for the parent to be able to discuss the child's traumatic experiences without extreme personal emotional distress—which is not helpful to the child or the parent(s).

TROUBLESHOOTING

How do you help kids to create trauma narratives when they are anxious and/or avoidant?

To minimize the level of avoidance from the start, it is important to present the idea of writing a narrative with a great deal of enthusiasm. For example, the therapist might emphasize the importance of deciding on a title and then starting the narrative with neutral or positive information (e.g., about self, a favorite activity, relationship with perpetrator before the trauma) Another approach that often helps reduce avoidance involves offering children a choice regarding the "chapter" to be written (e.g., "Would you like to write about when you told about the abuse or the first time the abuse happened?"). In general, we encourage therapists' creativity in finding effective ways of supporting children in overcoming their anxieties. Below are additional ideas and suggestions.

1. Ask for just one detail about the trauma ("Just tell me one thing.").
2. Agree on a certain amount of time to be spent on the trauma narrative ("only 5 minutes").
3. Plan a fun activity for the end of the session after working on the trauma narrative (e.g., telling jokes, sharing a talent).
4. Encourage positive self-talk (e.g., "I can do this"; "I was very brave for telling.").
5. Joke ("You don't remember *anything*? You gotta be kidding me. How dumb do you think I am?").
6. Emphasize that you know how hard it is to write this story ("I know that this can be hard, but you've shown such courage! I know you can do this.").
7. Praise ("You are one of the bravest kids I've ever known.").
8. Share your personal experience with trauma to model talking about it (if appropriate).
9. Use funky art techniques (we had a kid write the whole trauma narrative on a scarf; another agreed to write it on one of the author's [J.A.C.] arm but when she said it would be tough to photocopy, he agreed to go with paper).
10. Create the narrative with songs, colors, etc. Let the child pick a song, color, flower, animal, smell, etc., that describes a certain experience, then have him/her describe how it is like that smell, color, etc., while the therapist records what he/she says. Once the child starts to describe an episode, adding to it gets easier.
11. Use the computer to create the narrative and agree to 10 minutes of a computer game of the child's choice (within reason) after working on the trauma narrative.
12. Young kids: Let them show you what happened with dolls or puppets, then write it down and read it to them the next session, letting them correct/change your narrative so that it accurately reflects what happened.
13. Ask the child to explain what he/she thinks will happen if he/she talks about the trauma.
14. Praise the child for small steps, such as writing one sentence or talking about the trauma in the abstract.
15. Use the "riding the bike" analogy—"It's hard at first but gets

easier as you practice" (make sure the child can ride a bike first).

16. Do a "life narrative" instead of a "trauma narrative."
17. Use the Storybook Weaver Deluxe computer software program (available at www.kidsclick.com) and let the child make illustrations for each chapter written.
18. Let the child use window magic markers to create a "public service announcement" about the trauma.

It is important to remember that all of these strategies are designed to assist children with creating a narrative, *not* to elicit specific content. Children should be praised for whatever type of narrative they create; it is essential that the therapist not have any preconceived notions about the child's experience of the traumatic event. Some children who have multiple trauma histories may not include information about all the traumas they have experienced. Although the therapist should encourage the child with prompts to include the "worst moments," etc., the child ultimately needs to have the freedom to determine what should be included in his/her own narrative.

Do children ever start the narrative but stop in the middle?

It is very rare for children to refuse to finish the narrative in the middle. Sometimes they get bored with writing, however, and switching to drawing or another exposure-based activity can help. Usually children are excited to finish the narrative. They may need encouragement when they get to difficult sections, using the techniques described above. Also, it is important to emphasize to parents that treatment should not be interrupted or stopped while the child is creating the trauma narrative. Accordingly, if the family is unable to attend sessions for a period of time (e.g., a long vacation, financial issues), then the trauma narrative should not be started until after they return.

Can you tell us more about parents developing their own trauma narratives?

As we have noted previously, we have occasionally had parents develop their own narratives in parallel with their child's—that is, how they found out about their child's traumatic experience or how they learned of a traumatic family death. In these cases it is important to decide, using sensitivity, whether and how to share the parent's version with the child. In these instances (e.g., if the parent blamed him/herself for the child's abuse) sharing the parent's narrative would probably not be helpful for the child. Some parents, in their desire to ensure that they say everything they want to express, prepare a letter that they may share with their child after the child has shared the narrative. In such a letter, parents express their feelings of pride in their child and further clarify any points of confusion.

How do you do the trauma narrative with children in group homes or who otherwise have no parent in treatment?

For many children, the trauma narrative is the most difficult part of TF-CBT, so it is important to establish a source of support for these children that is available between treatment sessions if symptoms increase or trauma memories are triggered. In addition, the therapist can spend extra time making sure that such children "decompress" at the end of each session (e.g., practicing relaxation and other stress management skills prior to leaving). We have successfully used the TF-CBT model with many children who did not have parents involved in treatment, and they did not have more problems than children whose parents participated in treatment. It may be helpful to communicate with group home staff or other adults so that they are aware that children may need extra support and assistance during these segments of treatment.

Isn't there any concern that the trauma narrative will trigger worse PTSD symptoms in especially vulnerable patients, such as those with severe depression, multiple trauma histories, etc.?

We have actually found that the opposite is true. TF-CBT is superior to child-centered therapy (a treatment in which children do not directly discuss their trauma experiences) in resolving PTSD symptoms at the 1-year follow-up point for those children who had higher pretreatment scores on depression measures and those with a history of multiple traumas (Deblinger et al., 2005). Interestingly, in our most recent multisite study, many children who received the TF-CBT treatment said that the most helpful part was creating their trauma narratives. All of this evidence has convinced us that the trauma narrative is an important part of the TF-CBT model. We are currently conducting a multisite dismantling study of TF-CBT, which we hope will provide definitive answers to questions like this.

Cognitive Coping and Processing II
Processing the Traumatic Experience

After the child has created the trauma narrative and spoken at length about the trauma(s), the therapist should begin to identify, explore, and correct the child's trauma-related cognitive errors (i.e., inaccurate or unhelpful thoughts). *Inaccurate cognitions* are thoughts that are either absolutely false (e.g., "It's my fault my father got mugged because he was walking me to my friend's house when it happened.") or are so unrealistic as to approach impossibility (e.g., "I should have known that my new babysitter was a sexual abuser.") Unhelpful cognitions may also be inaccurate (such as the preceding two examples) or may be unhelpful despite being accurate (e.g., "People who get burned in a fire are in terrible agony.") or possibly accurate (e.g., "My mother must have been terrified before she was stabbed to death.").

Inaccurate cognitions sometimes articulate rescue or hero fantasies (wishing to have saved oneself or others from harm, often through the use of magical or super powers) and may arise, in part, from over-identification with real-life rescuers or heroes (e.g., firemen, police) depicted in the media. In other situations, inaccurate cognitions may reflect the child's attempt to gain mastery over the uncontrollable. Such an attempt is a common response to posttrauma fears that the world is unpredictable and dangerous. However, gaining a sense of control at the cost of blaming oneself for uncontrollable or unpredictable events is rarely helpful in promoting optimal adjustment. The therapist may find it useful to explain the concept of *accident* to the child—that is, that some things just happen, with no malignant intent or fault having to be assigned. For example, the therapist might ask the child, "Why do you think people invented the word *accident*? Was it just another word for *someone's fault*?")

Accurate but unhelpful cognitions may be seen by the child or parent as "facing reality" or "accepting the truth"—that is, as something that is necessary to truly deal with the situation at hand. In fact, focusing on the most horrifying (unhelpful) realities or possible realities of the traumatic event is a *choice*, not a necessity, and doing so may impair the child's ability to cope optimally with the trauma and/or loss.

EXPLORING AND CORRECTING INACCURATE OR UNHELPFUL COGNITIONS

One way to identify and correct dysfunctional thinking is to reread the child's trauma narrative in session, with a focus on all of the thoughts the child expressed in it. As each thought is verbalized in the narrative, the therapist should explore with the child whether this thought is accurate and helpful. For example, a child who discovered her brother's body after he committed suicide by hanging wrote in her narrative, "It was my fault, I should have known he was going to do this." The following dialogue illustrates how to use cognitive processing to address this inaccurate self-blame.

THERAPIST: Can you see any thoughts in this paragraph that are not accurate or helpful?

CHILD: I guess that it was my fault. I know it wasn't exactly my fault, I just felt that way. . . .

THERAPIST: Saying it was your fault is a thought; the feeling you had was . . . ?

CHILD: Guilty, I guess. I felt guilty 'cause I didn't know he was going to hang himself.

THERAPIST: How could you have known?

CHILD: I don't know, I just should have, I guess.

THERAPIST: Please, help me understand. Are you saying there were signs, or warnings, or something obvious that your brother did or said that clearly told you he was planning to hurt himself, and you just ignored it? Is that what you mean?

CHILD: No, no, nothing like that. I mean, he was unhappy a lot, but he never said he would do that.

THERAPIST: So as far as you know, there were no obvious signs that this would happen, that he would do this?

CHILD: No, but I still should have known. I mean, he was my *brother*, and we were really close.

THERAPIST: So just because you were his sister, you should have always, every minute, been able to read his mind? Even when he didn't give you any hints about what he was thinking?

CHILD: Well, not read his mind. But doesn't being close mean you understand people really well?

THERAPIST: Let's think about that for a minute. Was he close to anyone else besides you? Did he have a best friend or something?

CHILD: Yeah, he was super close to his girlfriend, and he was close to my mom sometimes, but not always.

THERAPIST: So did your mom or his girlfriend know that he was going to do this?

CHILD: No, no one knew or we would have done something. He didn't tell anyone what he really thought. He kept it all inside himself (*begins to cry*).

THERAPIST: And how about the people who are trained to recognize when someone is suicidal, such as his therapist or doctor. Did either of them know ahead of time that he was going to try this?

CHILD: No, he never told either of them. My mom said it made him really mad that they kept asking him about that, so I guess he didn't tell them either.

THERAPIST: So if I'm understanding you, unless you were a mind reader or a psychic or something, there was no way you could have known that he was going to do this, right?

CHILD: No, I guess not. I just wish he had told me. I wish he would have trusted someone.

THERAPIST: I totally understand that. I wish he had been able to tell someone how bad he was feeling too. But sometimes people who are depressed can't or won't do that. He decided not to tell anyone, so no one could know. Not even you.

CHILD: I know. I just feel so sad.

The above example illustrates the progressive logical questioning technique used in cognitive processing to explore and correct inaccurate thoughts about self-blame in relation to the traumatic event. In contrast is an example of a trauma-related cognition that was possibly true but unhelpful. This child found himself suddenly surrounded by several male teens, from outside of his school, who told him they would kill him if he didn't give them his backpack and all of his money. When referred to treatment, this child was unable to attend school due to overwhelming anxiety about being accosted again. His recurrent thought was "Scary things happen at school—it's dangerous there."

THERAPIST: So you keep thinking that school is always scary and dangerous?

CHILD: I just don't think it, it *is* scary and dangerous. I'm never going back there again.

THERAPIST: I understand why you got scared; that was a very frightening experience to live through when it was happening.

CHILD: You got that right. I don't know why anyone goes there.

THERAPIST: Please help me understand. School is always a dangerous, scary place, 'cause every single day, something bad happens there, is that right?

CHILD: Not every day, just some days. But it could happen at any time.

THERAPIST: I'm kind of confused. How long have you been going to this school?

CHILD: This is my third year, and it's my *last*! I'm never going back there.

THERAPIST: Help me understand. Every day you've been there, something dangerous has happened there, right?

CHILD: Not every day, just once.

THERAPIST: You mean, you went there every day for 2 whole years, and nothing bad ever happened there until now?

CHILD: Yeah, but now it's not safe ever again.

THERAPIST: I'm still confused. From how you described it, it sounded like bad things happen so often there, they are just a part of that school, and it will never be safe there again. But now you're telling me that only one bad thing ever happened there that you know of, right? So help me understand—how is this school so dangerous?

CHILD: It wasn't before, it just feels that way now.

THERAPIST: So it's not the school itself that's scary, it's something that was different that day from every other day you went there, right? What made the school so scary that day?

CHILD: Those punks stealing my stuff made it scary. And then they threatened me.

THERAPIST: Oh, so it was those guys, those four or five guys, not the school itself?

CHILD: Yeah, but there could be other guys like them there.

THERAPIST: And if there were, what do you think they would have learned from what happened to you? Do you think what happened to those guys—having to go to court and getting kicked out of school—is something other guys would like?

CHILD: No, I guess not.

THERAPIST: So the school is safe, it's those guys who were scary. And now they're gone, and any other guys are going to be worried about messing with you, 'cause you'll get them in big trouble.

CHILD: Yeah.

THERAPIST: I bet the other kids think you're pretty brave, like a hero or something, for standing up to those bullies.

CHILD: You think?

THERAPIST: Oh, yeah! I bet when you go back to school, kids will tell you they're glad you're back and no one will want to mess with you again.

CHILD: Well . . . maybe.

It is sometimes helpful to explore with the child the differences between bearing responsibility for a trauma and regret for an action taken or not taken. In some instances, children may have made active or passive decisions that increased their vulnerability to traumatization. For example, an adolescent who drinks excessively at a party, then accepts a ride home with boys she does not know well and is sexually assaulted by them, might blame herself for the assault. The therapist should help such an adolescent differentiate the regret she feels about drinking and taking a ride with strangers, from being responsible for the assault. This may be accomplished by using a similar "always" scenario as the one described above:

THERAPIST: So every girl who drinks and goes home with a stranger gets raped, right?

PATIENT: I don't think that always happens, but I deserved it for being so stupid.

THERAPIST: Wait. You mean there are some girls who have gotten drunk, been driven home by guys they didn't know well, and the guys didn't rape these other girls?

PATIENT: Yeah, that's happened to my friends. In fact, it's happened to me before.

THERAPIST: So even though drinking too much might not be a good idea, and riding home with guys you don't know is probably not wise, those things don't automatically mean you're going to get assaulted?

PATIENT: No, but they're still stupid.

THERAPIST: I agree they might not be the best decisions, and you regret that you did these things. But they are not what caused you to be assaulted. What had to happen for you to be raped, that happened this time but not the other times, and not to your friends?

PATIENT: The guys I was with were punks.

THERAPIST: So it was the guys who assaulted you who made it happen, who are responsible, right? You could have done exactly the same thing, and if they didn't decide to assault you, it wouldn't have happened.

PATIENT: That's true, but I still feel bad that I got drunk.

THERAPIST: It's OK to regret drinking—regretting a mistake is how we learn to make different choices in the future. However, that's very different from thinking that you were responsible for what those guys did to you.

Other common cognitive distortions children may have following a traumatic event include the following:

"I should have been able to keep it [the traumatic event] from happening."

"My family will never be OK again."

"It's my responsibility to become 'the man of the house' now that my dad is dead. "

"I will never get back to normal/never be happy again."

"The world will never be safe again."

"I can't trust anyone anymore."

"No one would like me if they knew about what happened in my family."

Once such distortions are identified (and new ones may develop or be verbalized for the first time at any point in therapy), cognitive-processing techniques should be employed to explore and correct them and to practice and reinforce more accurate and helpful thoughts.

COGNITIVE PROCESSING OF TRAUMATIC DEATH

Many children with traumatic grief struggle with cognitive distortions about the meaning and consequences of death resulting in body disfigurement, dismemberment, or fragmentation of body parts (including failure to ever make a positive identification of the loved one's remains, as was the case for most victims of the September 11th terrorist attacks, and as occurs in airline crashes, many war atrocities, and disaster situations. For example, in our experience some children believe that damaged, destroyed, or missing bodies continue to hurt even after death, or that loved ones whose remains are no longer intact become "haunted" or cannot go to heaven. Layne et al. (1999) described a "body reconstruction" technique that has been used with success in group therapy settings for adolescents in war zones (Layne, Pynoos, et al., 2001). This technique encourages the child to "put the body back together" for the loved one, through mental imagery and/or pictorial methods. Specifically, the child is encouraged to start by drawing a picture that depicts the body or body parts of the deceased that were present at the time of death or viewing. The child then adds on to this picture, either by drawing additional body parts, cutting and pasting additional body parts taken from magazine pictures, or mentally imagining these missing body parts being put back together to enable the body to be made whole again. When no remains are discovered (or when the body is present but disfigured), the child can place a photograph of the deceased (preferably a full-length picture taken when the deceased was in good health) in a prominent and easily visible place outside the coffin (R. Pynoos, personal communication, September, 2001). This technique, which has been used for many years in hospice settings, allows the child's last visual memory to be one of happier times.

Other children may need to "fix up" or repair the damaged body in their minds by writing, acting out, or imagining scenes whereby the body is taken to the hospital and sewn up, etc. Through these techniques, the child can thus be left with a mental image of the deceased as once again having an intact (albeit no longer living) body. In some cases in which no body remains are identified, we have found it helpful to provide the child with a copy of the official death certificate as a concrete confirmation of the physical reality of the loved one's death. It may be helpful to ask the child directly, "What would make your mother's death more real for you?" and then, if possible, following through on the child's suggestion. Of course, it is also important to educate the child that the state of one's corpse does not affect whatever happens after death. Some children may believe this information more readily if it is explained to them by a member of the clergy rather than a parent or therapist. Parents should be encouraged to ask their clergy for assistance in this way when it appears to be an issue for particular children.

In addition to self-blame for the traumatic event, intrusive horrifying thoughts about the agony and suffering experienced by the loved one prior to death, and misconceptions or frightening thoughts about death accompanied by disfigurement, may need to be addressed in sessions.

PROCESSING THE CHILD'S TRAUMA WITH PARENTS

In parallel with the child sessions, while discussing the trauma and/or sharing the child's trauma narrative with the parent, the therapist may have identified cognitive errors (inaccurate or unhelpful thoughts) that the parent has regarding the traumatic event and/or the child's behavior with regard to the trauma. The parent may also have developed cognitive distortions about the child's or his/her own response to the traumatic event. Common parental errors in this regard include the following:

"I should have known this would happen and kept my child safe."
"My child will never be happy again."

"Our family is destroyed."
"My child's life is ruined."
"I can't handle anything anymore."
"I can't trust anyone anymore."
"The world is terribly dangerous."
"My child can never recover from this."

The parent can be asked to share any troubling feelings or thoughts he/she may have had during the past week concerning the trauma his/her child suffered. The therapist then should ask the parent to examine his/her own thoughts for both accuracy and helpfulness. For example, with regard to the thought "My child will never be happy again," the reality is that most children will experience moments of normal mood or happiness even when suffering from PTSD or other serious emotional problems. The therapist may have personally witnessed a moment or two when the child was smiling, cheerful, or interacting normally with others. The therapist can point this out to the parent and ask whether there have been any other moments, however, fleeting, in which the child has seemed less sad. Once the parent is able to acknowledge that the child has experienced such moments, the therapist can point out that this shift to a lighter mood occurred even early in the trauma recovery process, when most children are distressed. Next the therapist can point out that "never" is a long time and that the child has already made a lot of progress and will continue to improve over time. Modifying the original inaccurate thought to a more realistic assessment (e.g., "My child is often sad now, but this is normal; even now she has moments of happiness, and as time passes, she will continue to get better.") will help the parent to feel more hopeful. This modification may also help the parent to offer encouragement to the child when the child is making similar distorted comments about him/herself.

The therapist might then discuss with the parent examples of some distorted thoughts the child gave in his/her parallel session and how cognitive-processing techniques were used to replace these distortions with more accurate and helpful thoughts. The parent should then be asked to come up with examples of how he/she has been thinking about the traumatic event, and to use the cognitive triangle to understand the impact of those thoughts on his/her feelings and behaviors. The therapist can model the cognitive-processing techniques and have the parent practice challenging his/her own inaccurate or unhelpful thoughts. Finally, the therapist can give the parent examples of cognitive distortions the child might make in the future, and have the parent practice how to effectively challenge these and help the child generate more accurate and helpful cognitions in this regard.

Most CBT interventions include the use of homework—that is, assignments of skills for the parent to practice between sessions; the skills are then discussed and fine-tuned with the therapist in subsequent sessions. As noted earlier, one of these assignments might be to track inaccurate or unhelpful thoughts the parent has between sessions and to change these thoughts to more accurate or helpful ones.

TROUBLESHOOTING

What can be done when the parent blames the child for the trauma?

It is important to process whether the parent has any realistic basis for blaming the child. Did the child, in fact, contribute in some way to his/her victimization? Would exploring the issues of responsibility versus regret be helpful in this regard? If the child had no responsibility whatsoever, it would be important to ascertain possible sources for the parent's blame of the child: Is this projection of the parent's own self-blame? If so, this projection should be explored in as nonjudgmental a manner as possible. Ultimately, if parental blame of the child is sufficiently detrimental to him/her, the negative impact would need to be addressed directly by the therapist and possible remedies discussed, including, if necessary, out-of-home placements (in the most extreme instances).

What if the child blames the parent for the traumatic event? What if the parent was, in fact, partly responsible?

This is a very difficult situation which needs to be addressed honestly with parent and child. One of the common scenarios in which this child blaming occurs is domestic violence, wherein the mother may return repeatedly to an abusive partner, placing herself and her children at risk for ongoing abuse and exposure to violence. Helping the child understand how the mother's personal trauma symptoms contributed to her decision making may be quite complex, especially if the child is young. Helping the mother make amends and assure the child that she will keep him/her safe in the future may be important steps in healing the relationship between the child and parent. Efforts to completely erase the mother's feelings of responsibility for remaining in the abusive relationship may not be the best course, because such efforts may inadvertently contribute to the mother's sense of powerlessness to escape now. At the same time, blaming the mother for her own personal victimization will certainly be unproductive for both mother and child. A better course of action is to assist the mother in understanding the dynamics of intimate partner violence (usually through referral to her own therapist) while encouraging mother and child to develop a safety plan together that assures the child's and mother's safety in the future (see Trauma-Focused Component 10 for more details).

In Vivo Mastery
of Trauma Reminders

Creating the child's trauma narrative is one method of helping the child to master his/her traumatic memories. However, narrative techniques alone may be insufficient to resolve generalized avoidant behaviors. As described earlier, some children have developed generalized fears that interfere with their ability to function optimally due to ongoing avoidance of perceived trauma cues *that are inherently innocuous.* Use of *innocuous* adds a very important distinction. It is usually adaptive to avoid situations that present ongoing threats to safety. For example, if a child is still being physically abused when he/she goes to her father's house, it is appropriate and healthy to want to avoid visiting the father. Therapists should not try to desensitize such a child to this trauma cue, because it serves as an "alarm" or "danger" signal that functions to keep the child safe. A similar example involves situations of ongoing domestic violence or community trauma, where it is important for children to be appropriately aware of antecedents to violence so that they can remove themselves from imminent danger and, if possible, alert the proper authorities to intervene. Attempting to desensitize such children to these cues or help them "master" them in a manner such that they do not respond with appropriate levels of anxiety and vigilance would endanger them rather than protect them.

In contrast, if the feared trauma cues are innocuous reminders of experiences that are in the past, they do not serve the purpose of maintaining safety in the present, and if overgeneralized, may interfere with healthy adaptation. A child who was sexually abused in the bedroom of her old home, and may be unwilling to sleep in the bedroom of a new home because this bedroom also reminds her of the sexual abuse, is an example of a fear that has generalized to an inherently innocuous cue (a bedroom where nothing bad has happened to her) that is disrupting the child's ability to regain a normal developmental trajectory (being able to sleep alone in her own room). In another situation, a child whose mother has been battered by her father is afraid to go to school, even though the father is in prison, because she may be afraid that something bad will happen to her mother if left alone. *In vivo* exposure is an intervention designed to gradually overcome this type of avoidance and thereby allow the child to regain optimal functioning.

One problem with avoidance is that it is very powerfully self-reinforcing. In other words, the more you avoid something, the more you come to believe that avoidance is the only possible way of coping with your fear. Conversely, the most powerful and effective way to overcome avoidance is through *not* avoiding, or exposing yourself to the very thing of which you are afraid. When the exposure to the feared situation does not result in the feared consequences, the anxieties associated with the once-avoided situation begin to diminish. This diminishment allows you to overcome your fear and learn that the more you face it, the less scary it becomes.

However, *in vivo* exposure requires an initial leap of faith that many children, parents, and therapists never make. The result of *not* facing the fear is that children are left unnecessarily, and sometimes tragically, to struggle for years with fears and avoidant behaviors they could have mastered long ago. The worst thing that the therapist can do is to start *in vivo* exposure and then stop in the middle because of a lack of belief in the intervention. If you do not believe it can work, it is better not to start it than to stop in the middle, because the lesson children will learn from this is that the fear is even stronger than they *and* you thought it was. You must be willing to persist, and the parent must be willing to persist, until the child has mastered the task and learned that he/she can tolerate what he/she fears. This is the same intervention that is used for treating school refusal in children and phobias in adults. It is known to be highly effective when used consistently. Here is how it works.

As is the case when creating the trauma narrative, the goal is not to overwhelm or flood the child with the feared situation or trauma reminder. Rather, the goal is to help the child gradually, a little bit at a time, get used to the feared situation so that each step is tolerable. By the end of the intervention the child should be able to be in the situation without undue anxiety or fear, because he/she has adapted to it a little at a time. The first step is to identify the feared situation. Let's use the case described above, of the child whose mother was battered and who now avoids leaving her mother alone for fear that something bad will happen. In developing an *in vivo* exposure plan, it is important to get as much information as possible about the most feared situations. It turns out that this child is able to leave the house, for example, to visit relatives or friends for a few hours on the weekend or in the evening. Her real fear is being at school, where she would not be able to call her mother on the telephone to check on her. Thus, in designing the *in vivo* exposure plan, the goal is for this child to be able to go to school all day without having to call her mother.

In order to design an effective plan, it is essential for the mother to be actively involved, comfortable, and in agreement with the plan. For example, if this mother were invested in keeping her child at home (e.g., to help care for younger siblings, help with housework, for emotional support), the intervention would be unlikely to succeed. The mother will need to reassure the child that the mother is able to keep herself safe, that nothing bad is going to happen to her, that she doesn't need or want the child at home to protect her, that the child's job is to get an education, and that this is how the child can best help the mother. If the mother has given the child contradictory messages in the past, it is important for the mother to assure the child that things are different now. Once the stage has been set to assure the child of her mother's safety, a plan should be agreed upon between mother, child, therapist, and the school regarding how to ease the child back into school. Depending on how much the child has attended school up to this point, the goal will be to progressively increase her exposure to school and being away from mother/home. Let's assume the child has been unable to stay at school for more than an hour on any day for the past month and has been allowed to come home "sick" each day at that time. Here is a sample plan for this child's *in vivo* exposure:

Week 1

Stay in school for 2 hours Monday and Tuesday,
3 hours Wednesday and Thursday,
4 hours Friday without calling home.
If the child gets sick, she may go to nurse's office for 5 minutes to practice breathing and relaxation. May call mother once during the day if the child stays longer than required time.
Each day the child reaches her goal, she gets a star; if she surpasses her goal, she gets two stars. Can watch movie(s) with Mom over the weekend: 5 stars = 1 movie rental, 10 stars = 2 movie rentals.

Week 2

Stay in school for 4 hours Monday,
5 hours Tuesday and Wednesday,
6 hours Thursday and Friday.
Same plan as above with regard to nurse's office, calling home, and
  rewards.

Week 3

Stay in school all day.
Same plan as above.

Week 4

Stay in school all day.
Same plan as above.

Each day when the child comes home from school, the mother must provide praise and reassurance as well as promptly producing the stars, if earned. It is also helpful if the teacher, school nurse, and counselor are made aware of the situation and provide support, reassurance, and reinforcement of relaxation exercises if utilized while in school.

In vivo exposure reliably changes most avoidant behaviors, which in itself has value for children's and families' adaptive functioning. However, we believe that the most important outcome of this intervention is that children regain a sense of their own competence and mastery. Feeling (and being) at the mercy of overwhelming fears is a disempowering experience. By learning that they can overcome their terrifying memories and fears, children gain self-efficacy that can have far-reaching positive consequences in their lives.

TROUBLESHOOTING

How do you reconcile confidentiality with informing the school of the plan to get children back to school?

The school does not need to know the details of the child's treatment to understand the plan for helping him/her return to school. The therapist should talk with the mother and child about what should and should not be shared with the school personnel regarding the treatment plan. There is typically no need to tell school personnel details about the nature of the child's traumatic experience.

*What if the parent wants to keep the child home, that is, depen-
dent. How can the therapist deal with that attitude?*

Many times the child is ready to grow up, and it is the parent who is
afraid to allow the child to move on and regain a normal developmental
trajectory. Discussing this issue in a supportive way with the parent can
be helpful, but many parents are unaware of their own needs to keep
their children in a younger stage of development and will insist that it is
the child who is unable to move forward. This is a difficult situation that
is unlikely to respond to behavioral interventions because the parent is
likely to undermine these. Helping parents to identify and acknowledge
their own underlying fears, both for their children and themselves, can
often be useful. The processing exercises described in Trauma-Focused
Component 7 can then be employed to dispute any dysfunctional
thoughts and beliefs. In addition, if the parent is not already engaged in
his/her own individual therapy, this may be the appropriate time for
such a referral.

TRAUMA-FOCUSED COMPONENT 9

Conjoint Child–Parent Sessions

The TF-CBT model includes conjoint sessions in which the child and parent meet with the therapist to review educational information, read the child's trauma narrative, and engage in more open communication. These sessions are intended to enhance the child's comfort in talking directly with the parent about the traumatic experience as well as any other issues the child (or parent) wants to address. Conjoint sessions typically occur after the child and parent have completed cognitive processing of the child's trauma experiences in individual sessions with the therapist. The therapist and family should decide together whether joint sessions are needed earlier in treatment or whether there should be relatively fewer or more conjoint sessions than individual sessions. For many families, it is easier to begin conjoint sessions with the practicing of skills (e.g., mutual praise) and/or more general discussions about the trauma (e.g., playing a question-and-answer game in which parents and children compete to see who knows more general information about the trauma experienced). This tactic allows them to experience immediate comfort talking about the trauma in the abstract and prepares them for reading and reviewing the trauma narrative together.

For 1-hour sessions, the joint sessions are typically divided so that the therapist first meets with the child for 15 minutes, then with the parent for 15 minutes, and finally, with the child and parent together for 30 minutes. The therapist should be flexible in adjusting this division of time to each individual family's needs.

If the goal of the joint session is to share the child's narrative, prior to having each set of joint sessions, the child should have completed the trauma narrative, be comfortable reading it aloud and discussing it in therapy with the therapist, and be willing to share it with the parent. The parent should have heard the therapist read the complete trauma narrative in previous individual parent sessions, be able to emotionally tolerate reading the trauma narrative (i.e., without sobbing or using extreme avoidant coping mechanisms), and be able to make supportive verbalizations when practicing responses during parent therapy sessions. In some instances, the therapist may need to review the child's narrative with the parent several times in order to help him/her gain sufficient emotional composure for the joint sessions to be productive. In addition, the therapist should role-play this interaction with the parent to ensure that his/her responses to the child are supportive and appropriate.

When the parent seems emotionally prepared to review the narrative with the child, the therapist should begin to work individually with the child to prepare him/her. The therapist should have the child read the trauma narrative out loud in individual sessions and suggest that the child is ready to share it with the parent. (The therapist should have already mentioned, at previous trauma narrative sessions, that sharing the narrative with the parent might occur.) The therapist should then suggest that the child write down questions or items that he/she would like to discuss with, or ask, the parent. These questions may pertain to trauma-related or other content about the child's traumatic experience which the child would like to be able to talk with the parent about more openly. Some examples include how the parent feels about the person who perpetrated the trauma; the parent's feelings or thoughts about the trauma; or any other questions about the traumatic event or family relationships the child may have. The therapist should have the child discuss these matters in this individual setting and assist him/her in formulating clear questions.

During the individual session with the parent (15 minutes before the joint session), the therapist should once again read the child's trauma narrative to the parent to ascertain that the parent is prepared to hear the child read the book directly to the parent. The therapist should then go over the child's questions with the parent and assist him/her in generating optimal ways of responding. The parent may also have questions for the child, and the therapist should help the parent phrase these in appropriate ways.

During the joint family session, the child should read the trauma narrative he/she has written to the parent and therapist. At the conclusion, the parent and therapist should praise the child for his/her courage in writing this trauma narrative and being able to read it to the parent.

The child should then be encouraged to raise issues of concern from the list prepared earlier, taking time to discuss each issue to the satisfaction of both parent and child. If the parent has also prepared questions for the child, these should be asked after the child has completed his/her questions. The therapist's role in this interchange should be to allow the child and parent to communicate directly with each other, with as little intervention as possible from the therapist. If either the child or parent has difficulty, or if either expresses an inaccurate or unhelpful cognition that the other does not challenge, the therapist should intervene (if judged clinically appropriate), so that the cognition does not go unquestioned. The therapist should also praise both the parent and child for completing the trauma narrative and joint family session components of treatment with such success.

At the end of this joint session, the therapist, parent, and child should decide on the content of the joint session to occur the following week. Often the child and parent have enjoyed this session so much that they are enthusiastic about having another and want to raise more issues to talk about together. If there was awkwardness or difficulty in communication, they may be less positive about the idea, but in this situation, the therapist should actively encourage another joint session in order to improve the parent's and child's comfort with talking about these subjects. The joint sessions may also be used to provide and reinforce psychoeducation about the child's trauma-related symptoms, the specific type of traumatic event the child experienced, etc.

Other activities in which families typically engage during joint sessions include talking about (1) attributions regarding the traumatic experience; (2) safety planning; (3) healthy sexuality in the case of sexual abuse; (4) healthy relationships; (5) anger resolution and picking appropriate romantic partners for teens who have been exposed to domestic violence situations; (6) conflict avoidance; (7) drug refusal and risk reduction strategies for children living in violent communities; and (8) sharing of emotional reactions to the child's traumatic experience (and, when appropriate, the parent's own traumatic reactions) and how these have changed during the course of therapy. Parents are understandably concerned for their future when children have gone through traumatic events, especially when parents observe changes in their children's emotions, cognitions, behaviors, and bodies subsequent to these experiences. Joint therapy sessions allow parents to overcome these concerns in constructive ways. Often parents are reassured when their children are able to discuss these issues openly with them in therapy and later at home. Bringing these concerns into the open also allows children to raise questions about areas that may have gone unaddressed in the family previously. For example, one adolescent girl who had witnessed her father attempt to strangle her mother was invited, during joint sessions, to talk about how to choose a nonabusive romantic partner for herself in the future. This discussion allowed her, for the first time, to openly express her negative feelings about her mother's new paramour, who, like her father, was prone to unpredictable rages during which he would start screaming "over nothing." When the mother pointed out that this man had never been physically violent, the girl responded, "Not yet. I don't want the first time to be him hurting you." This statement allowed the mother to comprehend the impact her current boyfriend's behavior was having on her daughter and led to her making changes that helped the daughter feel safer at home and better able to talk openly with her mother.

Therapists should expect that joint sessions will not always be easy or fun; growth and change can be difficult for children and parents. As new areas are discussed for the first time, old wounds, hurt feelings, misunderstandings, and miscommunications may be reopened. Working through these issues may not be painless for families, but it can be very rewarding. Therapists should use their clinical judgment to determine how many sessions should be spent on these issues, depending on how closely related they are to the child's traumatic experiences and current symptoms and how relevant to the child's family's present functioning. It can be helpful to end joint sessions on a positive note by actively encouraging parents and children to praise one another for something that they did in session or during the past week that was appreciated.

TROUBLESHOOTING

What if the child doesn't want to share the narrative with the parent, and the therapist agrees that this is not a good idea?

If the therapist believes that the parent will be unable to tolerate hearing the child's narrative or unable to appropriately support the child, it is probably better not to share the narrative with the parent. The joint sessions can be used instead to encourage other positive interactions between the child and parent. The therapist should offer a variety of cooperative activities to the child and parent in this regard and encourage them to engage in communication skill building through these activities.

How should conjoint sessions be managed if multiple siblings are being treated?

Typically, each sibling receives his/her own conjoint session with the parent(s). This format allows each child to share his/her own version of the traumatic experience(s) and to contextualize the experience in his/her own way. There may be some circumstances in which siblings want to share their narratives with one another; the therapist should facilitate this activity if parents are in agreement and it seems clinically indicated. Children can be given instructions to edit their narratives to make them more developmentally appropriate to share with younger siblings, if they would like to do so. It is surprising how instinctively children know what to edit, but therapists can always assist in this regard if they are unsure.

What if the parent becomes "negative" with the child during the joint session, that is, the parent is critical, etc.?

The therapist should try to model positive interactions between the child and parent, building a bridge between the two whenever possible. If the conjoint session becomes too negative, the therapist should end it and meet alone with the parent to explore what went wrong. However, if possible, the therapist should try to "shape" the parent's behavior more positively during the joint session.

Enhancing Future Safety
and Development

Children who have experienced trauma may suffer anxieties and concerns regarding their safety. Fears of innocuous trauma reminders (e.g., trauma memories, darkness) most often can be resolved through trauma narrative and processing work or through *in vivo* exposure tasks. However, other realistic safety concerns may best be addressed through education and training in safety skills. Unfortunately, we cannot and should not assure children that they will never suffer trauma again, but we can respond to children's fears by teaching them skills that will increase their feelings of self-efficacy and preparedness. In addition to teaching children standard safety precautions, such as looking both ways when they cross the street and wearing bike helmets and seat belts when traveling, there are many other safety lessons that are valuable to teach all children. These lessons are particularly important to share and/or review with children who have experienced trauma, because of the increased sense of vulnerability they may experience.

A child, for example, who was caught in a house fire may never be faced with this type of trauma again, but we cannot assure him/her of that. However, we can encourage a realistic view with regard to the likelihood of a fire recurrence and simultaneously enhance his/her feelings of safety by reviewing and practicing standard fire safety precautions (www.usfa.fema.gov/kids/flash.shtm). This facet of treatment would include talking about the importance of installing smoke alarms and making sure they are working; identifying and practicing escape plans (with at least two exit strategies from every room); staying low to the floor when escaping and getting out; calling 911; and *not* going back into the fire. A review of this information and practicing actual responses to fire can be incorporated into parent–child sessions as well as assigned for homework so that children get additional practice *in vivo*.

Just like fire safety, personal safety is important for all children to learn. However, it is particularly important for children who have suffered abuse or exposure to violence because they are at high risk for revictimization (Arata, 2000; Boney-McCoy & Finkelhor, 1995). Reviewing the above basic safety skills about seatbelts, crossing the street, and fire safety with children and parents may help to normalize the introduction of personal safety skills training while highlighting their importance.

The timing of teaching personal safety skills should be carefully considered; it is generally preferable to teach these skills after the youngster has completed much of his/her trauma narrative. This sequence reflects the fact that most children do not naturally react to trauma with what we would consider optimal responses. It is rare, for example, for children to assert themselves effectively enough to stop abuse or violence. Therefore, so as not to inadvertently undermine the child's comfort in sharing his/her real, but less than optimal, responses to prior traumatic experiences, it is best to postpone the teaching of safety skills until at least some of the narrative or other exposure work has been completed. When children are taught personal safety skills too early, they may feel guilty for not having utilized such skills to stop the violence or abuse, and they may incorporate these behaviors into their narratives to "look good." Gradual exposure and processing work is most effective when children report experiences *as they happened*. Later, as children are processing and making meaning of the experiences, they may want to explore alternative responses that may help keep them safe in the future.

A relatively early introduction of personal safety skills training, however, may be warranted if the child remains in a higher risk environment. This is sometimes the case for children who have been exposed to domestic violence. Although treatment typically would not begin until safety issues were addressed, some children will continue to have contact with individuals who have some potential for aggressive or even violent behavior. For example, when individuals leave spouses because of domestic violence, their spouses may retain visitation rights with the children. In such instances, even if they have never been physically harmed themselves, children will often continue to fear that parent's potential for violence toward them as well as others. This is a circumstance in which some level of personal safety training would be warranted relatively early in the process.

In general, before engaging children in safety skills training, it is important to acknowledge and praise their responses to previous traumas suffered. Although, as noted above, these responses may not have prevented the trauma, some aspect of how they responded was most likely productive and can be recognized with praise. In fact, most children can be praised for taking the most important step toward safety, which is telling someone about their victimization. The appropriateness of praise holds true even if the trauma was abuse that was discovered and reported by someone who witnessed it. Although in this case the child did not initially tell, he/she did find the courage to tell someone about it at some point (e.g., a police officer, a child protection worker, a therapist), and such a revelation also further serves to protect the child, as well as other children, from suffering similar abuse in the future. To reduce the likelihood that safety skills training will leave children feeling as if they didn't do the right thing in response to prior trauma(s), it is important to emphasize that they responded in the best way they knew how at that time. As a therapist, you might introduce this concept as follows:

THERAPIST: Most children never learn about what to do if someone is abusive or violent. We talk to kids about what to do in case there's a fire or other emergency in the home, but most often we don't teach children exactly what to do when someone is being abusive. So what you did when your dad was hitting your mom was the best way you knew how to respond at that time!

CHILD: I don't think so 'cause I didn't get help.

THERAPIST: Did anyone ever teach you what to do if your dad hit your mom?

CHILD: No.

THERAPIST: So it is not surprising that you didn't know exactly how to get help. But you did do something very helpful when you got your sister to stay by your side.

CHILD: I guess so.

THERAPIST: And what else did you do that was very brave?

CHILD: I don't know.

THERAPIST: What did you do when the child protection worker asked you about what happened?

CHILD: I told her what happened.

THERAPIST: Was that hard to do?

CHILD: *Really hard.* I didn't want to tell her anything 'cause I thought I might never see my dad again.

THERAPIST: So I think it was very brave of you to answer all her questions so clearly.

CHILD: I guess.

THERAPIST: Today we are going to practice some special skills that might help you if you are ever in a situation where you think you or someone else might be in danger. This doesn't mean that you did anything wrong before, because you did the best you could do at that time, especially since it was pretty scary, and no one ever told you what to do in that kind of situation.

CHILD: It was scary. But I'm not scared now!

THERAPIST: Great. So let's talk about some skills that might help you if you are concerned about someone's safety in the future.

CHILD: OK.

Children who have experienced multiple traumas, particularly in the area of interpersonal violence, may realistically fear the recurrence of violence or abuse. In fact, as noted above, there is considerable evidence that children who have suffered victimization or exposure to violence may be at high risk for revictimization in adolescence and adulthood. Thus, it is important to incorporate skill-building exercises that will reduce children's risk of future victimization and may enhance feelings of self-efficacy in facing potential future life stressors.

Several studies have clearly documented that parental involvement seems to enhance children's retention and utilization of personal safety skills (e.g., Finkelhor, Asdigian, & Dziuba-Leatherman, 1995; Deblinger et al., 2001). Therefore, while personal safety skills training may begin in individual sessions with children, it will be important to ultimately involve parents in the learning and practicing of these skills.

The first step in helping children keep themselves safe involves enhancing their ability to communicate with others about scary and confusing experiences. Children need to have the vocabulary, communication skills, and the confidence to respond effectively to abusive or traumatic experiences. Even for children, *knowledge is power*. Reviewing basic facts about sexual abuse and family and community violence not only provides children with knowledge but also helps them identify potential threats and may increase their likelihood of telling someone about abuse-related concerns or other disturbing experiences (e.g., being bullied, witnessing community violence). As indicated earlier, providing basic information about how many children experience abuse and/or are exposed to violence, how children feel in response to these experiences, and who might engage in aggressive behavior enhances children's understanding of the issues. It is again important to ensure that children have the language that they need to express both their feelings and their concerns. Practicing the sharing of feelings and teaching "doctors' names for private parts" establishes some basic skills for communicating all forms of victimization, including sexual abuse, which is often particularly difficult for children to disclose if they are not comfortable with the language required to describe their experiences. This type of psychoeducation can be provided via a variety of books, videos, and educational games.

In general, it is important to teach children about possible dangers in their environment as well as to encourage them to pay attention to their "gut" reactions and perceptions of danger. Children who have experienced violence in their lives and/or are suffering PTSD sometimes are less sensitive to danger cues because these cues may trigger PTSD responses that interfere with the effective processing of potential threats. For this reason it is important to have children rehearse how they might respond to potentially dangerous situations. These types of role plays not only help children develop safety skills, but, by means of habituation, may lead to reduced physiological and dissociative responses to threats. It is also important to note that children who have been exposed to violence repeatedly may be more likely to perceive danger where no such threat exists and thus may overreact to innocuous cues with aggressive responses. Again, role plays that help children imagine and act out scenarios they may face will give them opportunities to practice engaging in assertive responses rather than passive or aggressive responses. In sum, education, skill building, and experiential exercises may help children recognize and respond more effectively to real threats in the future.

It is important for parents and children to understand that although personal safety skills training does not guarantee the prevention of future victimization, the skills are likely to enhance children's feelings of control and confidence in responding to complex personal situations. In fact, there is some evidence that when children receive this type of training, they are more likely to disclose victimization attempts and/or utilize self-protection strategies (Finkelhor et al., 1995).

Important concepts to incorporate into personal safety skills activities include (1) communicating feelings and desires clearly and openly, (2) paying attention to "gut" feelings, (3) identifying people and places that provide safety, (4) learning body ownership (rules about "ok" and "not ok" touches), (5) learning the difference between secrets and surprises, (6) asking for help until someone provides the help needed.

Communicating feelings and desires is difficult to do in stressful situations, especially if it is not something that is typically done in comfortable, safe settings. Potentially difficult peer interactions can provide the context for initial role plays in which children can practice asserting themselves and communicating clearly and directly.

> THERAPIST: Today I would like to teach you some skills that can be helpful at school if someone says something nasty or bothers you in some way. Do you ever have experiences like that?
>
> CHILD: Sure. One kid bothers me all the time.
>
> THERAPIST: What does he do?
>
> CHILD: He calls me *slob*.
>
> THERAPIST: Why don't we act out what you do when he calls you slob. Can I be that boy just for a moment?
>
> CHILD: OK.
>
> THERAPIST (as boy): Hey, slob—what are you doing, making a big mess again?
>
> CHILD: What are *you* doing, fart face?
>
> THERAPIST: Now, what does Billy usually do when you say that?
>
> CHILD: He just yells "SLOB" louder and louder until everybody starts paying attention.
>
> THERAPIST: OK, well let's see if you can try a different response that might work better. Remember how we talked about "I" statements and telling someone really clearly how you feel and what you want them to do? This time I want you to stand tall and say "I feel _____ when you call me a slob. Don't call me that name anymore."
>
> CHILD: OK, I'll try.
>
> THERAPIST (as boy): Great. . . . Hey, "BIG SLOB," what are you doing now?

CHILD: I feel mad when you call me "BIG SLOB." Please don't call me that anymore.

THERAPIST: Wow! That was great. I really like how you expressed yourself so clearly and directly. Now let's try it one more time with that same strong tone of voice, but this time put your shoulders back and look me in the eyes when you say that.

As noted in the role play, in addition to coaching children in their verbal communication, it is also important to coach their nonverbal behavior. For example, after each role play, the child can be given positive feedback as well as gentle but specific constructive feedback on both verbal and nonverbal behaviors.

In addition to having children practice expressing their feelings in session, it is very helpful to have parents encourage effective feeling expression by shaping and praising their children's efforts to express their feelings at home. Parents can be encouraged to prompt feeling expression by asking their children more often how they feel. Parents sometimes find it difficult to respond effectively to their children's expressions of anger. For example, instead of responding defensively when a child says, "I'm mad at you, Mom," parents can be coached to say "Thank you for telling me you're mad. Would you like to talk about it?" This type of response often takes children by surprise and is much more likely to lead to a productive conversation while also reinforcing a behavior that is much more effective than kicking the wall or other behaviors in which children engage to express their anger.

Teaching children to pay attention to their "gut" reactions will help them recognize internal cues that signal a need to get away to a safe place and get help. Sometimes children automatically react to danger and their own physiological arousal by freezing rather than taking action. There may be some instances in which the freeze response can, in fact, be protective; nevertheless, it is important for children to identify places and people with whom they associate with safety so that they can get help as soon as possible thereafter. This step is particularly important when working with children who have been exposed to domestic violence. Parents are encouraged to help children develop a safety plan that should include self-protective strategies, the identification of places and people who can realistically provide safety and assistance, and encouragement to call 911 (Runyon, Basilio, Van Hasselt, & Hersen, 1998). As it is hard to know who might be accessible in any given situation, it helps to create a list of safe places and trustworthy people. Once again, simple role plays can help children practice these skills in individual sessions and later in conjoint sessions with their parent(s). Moreover, it is important to encourage parents to practice these skills with their children in their own home (with the caveat that phones should always be unplugged when practicing calling 911). In addition, others involved in the safety plan (e.g., a neighbor) should be informed and engaged in the practice role plays when possible.

> THERAPIST: Today I thought we could practice the safety plan we worked on with your mom last week.
>
> CHILD: OK.
>
> THERAPIST: Now let's make believe that when your dad drops you off from a visit, he and your mom start getting into one of those really bad fights they used to have. Can you tell me how you could tell that your mom is scared or might get hurt?
>
> CHILD: Usually mom starts to cry and yell.
>
> THERAPIST: OK. And then as your mom indicated, if she starts to yell *stop* and your father doesn't stop, what are you going to do?
>
> CHILD: I'm going to go into mom's bedroom and call 911.
>
> THERAPIST: Great. Let's practice that. I'll unplug this phone so you can dial.
>
> CHILD: OK. (*Dials 911.*)
>
> THERAPIST: 911—can I help you?
>
> CHILD: My parents are fighting and I'm afraid my mom is going to get hurt bad.
>
> THERAPIST (as 911 dispatcher): Where are you now—can you give me the address?
>
> CHILD: 19 Poplar Avenue.
>
> THERAPIST (as 911 dispatcher): Are you safe, where you are?
>
> CHILD: No, I'm scared. I'm going to go out the back door to our neighbor's house.
>
> THERAPIST (as 911 dispatcher): OK, the police are on their way. You can go to the neighbor's right now.

It is important for parents to be reminded that children can learn to be respectful to adults, while also understanding that sometimes even adults can say or do something that is wrong. This point is particularly important with regard to OK versus not OK touches. Again, personal safety education about child sexual abuse starts with a review of the information regarding what kinds of touches are, or are not, OK and the proper names of the private parts. Children can be reminded that when an adult or older child breaks the rules and uses not OK touching, or when the situation gives the child an uncomfortable feeling, it is important to try to say *NO*, then GO (i.e., get away) and TELL (i.e., report the inappropriate behavior to a responsible adult). With regard to sexual abuse as well as other victimization, children are often urged or threatened by perpetrators to keep these abusive interactions a secret. Teaching children the difference between secret surprises and scary secrets is important here: *Surprises* are secrets that kids don't keep forever and that are usually fun to share eventually (e.g., such as sharing a surprise gift or party); *scary secrets*, in contrast, are secrets that kids are asked to keep from their parents and/or never tell anyone about. These are secrets that kids don't want to keep, even if they told the person they would. Moreover, when revealing a scary secret such as sexual abuse, it is important for the child to persevere—to keep telling the secret—until he or she finds someone who understands and helps.

As noted above, there are many excellent books and videos (DVDs) that provide information about personal safety (see www.creative-therapystore.com). However, recent research suggests that children learn best through interactive discussion and role plays that test their understanding and internalization of the concepts presented (Finkelhor et al., 1995; Deblinger et al., 2001). A series of books and workbooks written by Stauffer and Deblinger (2003, 2004) provides an excellent framework for parents, teachers, and/or counselors with which to engage children in such discussions, while also providing ideas for role plays to practice personal safety skills (www.hope4families.com).

PART III

GRIEF-FOCUSED
COMPONENTS

Introduction to the
Grief-Focused Components

The PRACTICE components described thus far successfully allow most children with childhood traumatic grief to become "unstuck" from dwelling on the traumatic aspects of the nature of their loved one's death. These children can now begin to address the typical tasks of grieving described on page 16. It is important to recognize that grief is a process that can be long-lasting and, as such, we do not expect that children's grief will be "resolved" at the conclusion of this time-limited treatment model. However, we have found that once children have received help to become "unstuck" from the traumatic aspects of their loved one's death, their psychiatric and CTG symptoms abate, they experience improved adaptive functioning. In addition, parents who participate in this treatment also experience relief from their personal PTSD and depressive symptoms (Cohen, Mannarino, et al., 2004; Cohen et al., 2005).

Like the trauma-focused components, we view the grief-focused interventions of this model as a components-based hybrid approach that integrates grief-sensitive interventions (adapted from child treatment studies of children experiencing parental loss due to cancer [Christ, 2000; Siegel, Kraus, & Ravies, 1996; Siegel, Ravies, & Kraus, 1996] as well as writings by leading authorities in the grief and traumatic grief fields [Eth & Pynoos, 1985; Wolfelt, 1991; Fitzgerald, 1992, 1995;

Webb, 1993; Rando, 1993, 1996; Worden, 1996; Goldman, 1996, 2000; Nader, 1997; Black, 1998] and our own experience in treating bereaved children) and cognitive-behavioral principles. The specific components include grief psychoeducation, grieving the loss and resolving ambivalent feelings about the deceased; preserving positive memories of the deceased; and redefining the relationship with the deceased and committing to present relationships. Each of these is described in the following pages.

GRIEF-FOCUSED COMPONENT 1

Grief Psychoeducation

Even after they have talked about the traumatic aspects of the event, it may be hard for many children to talk about death. To some extent, this inability is modeled by adults, who often "do not know what to say" when someone dies, and as a result, may say nothing at all, or avoid the topic entirely.

GRIEF PSYCHOEDUCATION FOR CHILDREN

It may be helpful for these children to start the grief-focused portion of therapy by *reading a developmentally appropriate book about death*. Such books provide a model for children to talk openly about death, and many also educate readers about aspects of death and grief. Examples of this type of book are *Goodbye Mousie* (Harris, 2001), *I Miss You: A First Look at Death* (Thomas, 2001, for younger children), *When Dinosaurs Die: A Guide to Understanding Death* (Brown & Brown, 1996), and *What on Earth Do You Do When Someone Dies?* (Romain, 1999, for preteens and adolescents). We have found that children respond well to reading out loud in therapy, books written about situations like theirs, because doing so gently introduces them to talking about their own situation without requiring them to immediately talk about themselves. In this sense, reading such books is an initial, gradual form of exposure to death and grief.

Another option for introducing the general topic of grief is to play a grief-education game such as *The Good-Bye Game* (Childswork/Childsplay) or *The Grief Game* (Jessica Kinglsey Publishers). These games ask "neutral" questions about death and mourning (e.g., "What is a funeral?") rather than specific questions about a personal loss.

Next the therapist can ask the child to draw a picture of what he/she thinks happens when someone dies (Stubenbort et al., 2001). Although some misconceptions about death may have been addressed in the trauma-focused interventions discussed previously (i.e., body reconstruction), the child may still have many confusing ideas about death. The therapist should correct these in a manner that is consistent with the family's cultural and religious beliefs (as discussed in the following section). The therapist may then ask the child to list different feelings that kids or grownups might have when someone they love dies. The "Color Your Life" technique can also be used to describe different feelings adults (not necessarily the child him/herself) might feel if someone died. Thus, in three steps (reading a book or playing a game about death, asking the child about his or her beliefs about what happens after death, and listing or drawing feelings that people may have following the death of a loved one), the child has gradually been exposed to, and tolerated, talking about death in the abstract. The next step is to encourage the child to talk directly about his/her own grief and to begin grieving the loss, as addressed in the following components.

GRIEF PSYCHOEDUCATION FOR PARENTS

In addressing grief-focused issues with the parent, it is important for the therapist to understand the parent's familial, religious, and cultural beliefs with regard to death, mourning, and grieving. Some of these issues may have been touched on in the trauma narrative parent component. As the grief-focused phase of the child's treatment begins, the therapist should discuss these issues again with the parent. In some instances, the parent may be struggling with conflicts between what his/her family/religion/culture dictates to be "normal" or "appropriate" grieving, and what he/she is actually thinking, feeling, or doing. For example, parents may feel negatively judged or rejected by their religious community if they no longer have faith in God; or a parent who begins to date again after a few months may feel that family and friends are angry about this "disrespect" for the deceased. Providing a nonjudgmental, accepting setting for the parent to discuss these issues may be of great benefit for both parent and child.

It is also important for the therapist to ascertain the parent's perception of the child's understanding of death. Often parents feel upset or confused because their children show very *little* emotion about the death of the loved one. This absence of affect may be due to shock, developmental limitations in the child's ability to comprehend the permanence of death, PTSD avoidance, or attempts by the child to shield the parent from knowing how upset he/she really is. Certain circumstances may also make it difficult for the child to believe that the loved one is dead or to know how to act. For example, for many days following the terrorist attacks on New York and Washington, DC in September 2001, thousands of people were shown on television posting pictures and descriptions of their loved ones, obviously holding out hope that they were still alive beneath the wreckage. Children who saw this coverage in the media or in person might well have been confused and may have believed, even months later, that their loved one was still alive. Even observing firsthand how the hope of the adults in their life turned gradually to grief may not have convinced such children that the "final" truth was known. In general, the younger the child, the more likely these kinds of circumstances are confusing. The parent may therefore need considerable help in understanding the child's concept of death, and may need assistance in providing age-appropriate explanations of death to the child. If the parent prefers that the therapist provide these explanations, the therapist and parent should discuss and agree ahead of time on what precisely the therapist will tell the child so that the explanation is consonant with the parent's belief system. In this way, information provided to the child by the therapist and parent will be similar and not cause further confusion in the child.

As noted above, although the TF-CBT treatment model focuses on addressing the child's trauma- and grief-related issues, it is likely that the parent will also address his or her own trauma and grief issues, to some extent, in this treatment. It is expected that hearing about the child's grieving process during therapy will trigger the expression of some of the parent's own grieving. We believe that assisting the parent in resolving personal emotional distress is likely to have a positive impact on the child's response to treatment. Thus the therapist should encourage the parent's expression of feelings related to the death of the loved one and assist him/her in addressing and, to some extent, resolving personal grief issues. As the parent becomes more comfortable with discussing these feelings (including ambivalent feelings about the deceased if these are present), he/she will model for the child that it is OK to talk about death and the deceased loved one, even to express negative feelings. This process culminates in the joint sessions at the end of therapy, which are discussed in the last section, "Treatment Review and Closure." Typically, the parent's personal grief issues have some commonalities with the child's issues, but there are also differences due to the different relationship the parent had with the deceased, as well as the fact that the parent is an adult. Child-focused parental grief interventions are described in Grief-Focused Component 2. Regardless of the parent's own grief issues, the therapist should emphasize the importance of the parent expressing his/her feelings to the child in an appropriate manner (i.e., the parent does not necessarily tell the child everything he/she discusses with the therapist).

Providing psychoeducation to the parent about the "normal" grieving process—that is, that there is no "normal" process for the profound pain associated with the loss of a partner or child—can be very helpful to parents. Several public websites are available in this regard; some of the most helpful are listed below:

- compassionatefriends.com
- www.dougy.org
- www.genesis-resources.com
- www.centerforloss.com

TROUBLESHOOTING

How can there be no "normal" grieving? How can we provide psychoeducation if there is no information about what is normal?

Accepting that there is a very broad range of "normal" with regard to grieving the loss of a loved one is very difficult for some therapists but is also very important. Of course, as mental health professionals, we have some parameters for clinical concern. For example, active suicidality is cause for concern in our eyes, even if some would consider it within the realm of "normal."

What is the difference between bereavement, grief, and mourning?

Bereavement is the state of having lost a loved one to death. Grief is the emotional distress related to the loss of a loved one. Mourning is the range of cultural rituals associated with death.

What do you think about sharing personal grief experiences with families?

Again, this is a personal decision. Unlike trauma histories, grief is fairly universal in that most people have experienced a familial death or the loss of a close loved one at some point, and there is much less social stigma attached to most deaths than to many traumas. As with trauma histories, therapists should be clear about the reasons they are sharing personal histories of loss with children and parents, if they choose to do so, and weigh the potential benefits of such self-disclosure versus the potential harm. In any case, the focus should remain on the child's and parent's loss; therefore, we recommend that personal sharing be limited in terms of scope and detail. For example, one of us (J.A.C.) was treating a child whose infant sibling had died of sudden infant death syndrome (SIDS). The child's mother expressed the cognition, "Everyone looks at me like maybe I caused my baby's death. No one understands how devastated my daughter and I feel, how sad we both are." After the typical cognitive processing interventions proved to be unhelpful, I shared with the mother that when I was a child, my infant sister had also died suddenly. The mother responded, "Oh, so that's why you do this kind of work." The hoped-for result (i.e., that the mother would come to see that I could truly understand how she felt) did not occur. Rather, this self-disclosure ended up creating a distance between the mother and me. Unfortunately, therapist self-disclosure often leads to this outcome—i.e., clients may assume that therapists have "not worked out their own issues" and this is why they are working in the same area in which they have had previous personal traumatic experiences.

Grief is so related to religious and existential beliefs. Should the therapist answer these religiously oriented questions if children ask them (e.g., "Do you believe in God?").

This again depends on therapists' personal preferences. We tend to think that most children ask this type of question for a reason—that is, they are looking for a certain kind of answer. We would tend to answer first in a manner that would encourage the child to answer for him/herself (e.g., "That's a pretty big question. What do you think about God?"), but if pressed, would probably answer in a manner that is honest but as consistent with the child's or parents' views as possible. For example, a 6-year-old boy from a devout family whose family relied on their faith to help them through their trauma and grief told one of us (J.A.C.) that he "hated God." When he asked me whether I still go to church or if I was mad at God, I replied, "I haven't been to church lately, but I still pray to God and I believe he listens to us, even when we're mad at him. How about you?" The little boy wasn't sure about this answer, so I told him, "One of my favorite parts of praying is always the songs. So maybe you could just sing instead of pray what you want to say to God." He then started to sing "Yes, Jesus loves me, the Bible tells me so . . . ." Therapy should typically not devolve into a philosophical or theological debate.

Grieving the Loss
and Resolving Ambivalent Feelings
about the Deceased
"What I Miss and What I Don't Miss"

GRIEVING THE LOSS: "WHAT I MISS"

Grieving the loss includes grieving both the loss of the relationship with the deceased in the present (including all the fun, comforting, loving aspects of that relationship), and the loss of things that might have occurred in the future, but now will never be. These two dimensions are addressed separately in this discussion, but in therapy, they are often intermingled.

Grieving the loss of the relationship the child had with the loved one requires the child to remember, identify, and name the things the deceased and the child did with and for each other, which will no longer occur. These may include everything from basic caregiving (i.e., tasks that could be performed by a variety of other caretakers) to the most unique aspects of the relationship. Even mundane tasks such as cooking and cleaning may have been special to the child because of the unique way in which the deceased involved the child in their doing (e.g., a mother may have had the children each perform special tasks in baking cookies—one measured, one poured, one stirred—which made baking cookies more than a mere food preparation task). The therapist should encourage the child to describe these *special aspects of the relationship, which are now lost.* Some children may want to list things they miss in different categories, for example, as follows:

- "Things I miss doing with Mom"
- "Places I miss going with Mom"
- "Special rituals with Mom that I miss"

The child may also write the feelings that he/she previously experienced while sharing those activities or interactions with the deceased, then write how he/she feels now, knowing that those activities will not be shared with the loved one again, except in memory. Some children may choose to list these on a piece of paper, others may draw pictures, make a collage, or use other creative techniques to express what they miss. This activity is expected to prompt sadness, which is part of the normal grieving process. The therapist should explain to the child that almost everyone feels this great sadness after losing a loved one, and that it is a natural result of having loved the person so much. It may be helpful for some children to know that other family members are also sad and missing the things they used to share with the deceased; however, children who feel overly protective of remaining family members may not benefit from hearing about their grieving.

In addition to losing the past relationship with the deceased, children have also *lost things that might have occurred in the future*, which can now never be shared with the deceased. Important rites of passage—confirmation, high school graduation, weddings, birth of one's first child—are times usually shared with family and other loved ones. The absence of a parent or other loved one at such events is a significant loss to many children. Less celebrated but nonetheless meaningful events occur throughout the course of children's growing-up years—being in a school play, participating in sports competitions, getting academic or extracurricular prizes—these are all events at which children hope to have their parents and other loved ones present. Recognizing, naming, and grieving these losses are also important for many children and should be included in the discussion of what has been lost, along with the feelings that accompany the naming of these losses.

Preparing for the loved one's absence at these events is one manner in which children can come to realize that in the future there may be many reminders of the loss. *Anticipating "loss reminders"* (Layne et al., 1999) and developing positive coping responses to address them are two areas children can start to address in therapy. It is hoped that this preparation together with their trauma-focused work treatment (i.e., writing the narrative and participating in other exposure exercises) will make them less vulnerable to being overwhelmed when such reminders occur in the future. One approach to this exercise is to ask children to think of ways in which these events could be made special despite the absence of the loved one. Some children "dedicate" their special events to the deceased in some manner, either publicly or privately. For example, one young man announced that his bar mitzvah was "in honor of my sister, who is still with me in spirit"; some adolescents run a big race or play an important game "for my dad"; others invite someone special to these events in lieu of the deceased, such as the deceased's best friend; a teenage girl whose father died months before her high school graduation wrote, "I will be happy because I will remind myself of how proud my dad would be of me if he could be there." Children may also want to list these in the following manner:

Things I will miss in the future: How I will cope:

_____   _____

_____   _____

_____   _____

_____   _____

Grieving these losses will not be accomplished in a single treatment session or, indeed for many children, even in the course of several weeks of therapy. The goal is not to complete the grieving process during therapy but to model for children that it is OK to feel great sadness when they have experienced a great loss, to give them an opportunity to express these sad feelings in a setting where they do not have to worry about others' vulnerability, and to encourage them to believe that their pain will diminish over time.

RESOLVING AMBIVALENT FEELINGS
ABOUT THE DECEASED: "WHAT I DON'T MISS"

It is often difficult to acknowledge imperfections in a loved one who has died. This difficulty may be intensified if the death occurred in a sudden, unexpected, traumatic manner, which sometimes leads to the deceased being viewed as a martyr or hero by the child or others. However, there may also be "unfinished business" between the child and the deceased— unresolved conflicts or words said or unsaid that are now regretted by the child.

This ambivalence may be most apparent in situations where the deceased was somewhat responsible for his/her own death (e.g., a death caused by suicide or drug overdose, a "drug deal gone bad," or an accident in which the loved one was driving while intoxicated). In these situations, the child has to deal with the *stigma* associated with these activities in addition to trauma and grief issues. In fact, one of the main differences we have seen between children who lost a loved one to a highly publicized disaster (e.g., airline attack, bombing, terrorist attack) and those who lost their loved one to interpersonal violence, accidents, or suicide is this issue of stigma. In the former case the deceased are seen as innocent victims, if not heroes, and there is typically an outpouring of public attention, emotional support, and often public and/or government financial assistance. These children are often rightfully proud of their fallen loved one, and this positive aspect is often helpful in resolving the trauma/death issues. However, these positive aspects are rarely present for the second group of children, whose loved one died in less "heroic" circumstances. In these situations there may be strong extended family support but insinuations or innuendos in the broader community. Even children whose parents were murdered by strangers are often faced with questions about whether the deceased was somehow partly responsible for his/her own demise (e.g., they may hear adults or peers say, "You have to wonder what she was doing in that neighborhood so late at night.") If these issues have not been addressed in the trauma-focused portion of therapy, they may arise when discussing "unfinished business" in the relationship with the deceased.

Regardless of the type of trauma that led to the loved one's death, almost all children have occasional conflicts with their siblings or parents, and these may have been unresolved at the time of the death. Adolescents, in particular, might have gone through weeks or months of thoughtless, rude, or rebellious interactions with the loved one—conflicts not resolved prior to the death. This lack of resolution typically leads to guilt feelings in the surviving child, but may also leave the child with unresolved resentment or anger, which remains unspoken due to family or social expectations to "not speak ill of the dead." After giving the child an opportunity to discuss these issues and feelings, the therapist should normalize them by pointing out that all children have conflicts with their parents/siblings at times, but typically these are discussed and worked out over time. The therapist can then suggest that although the premature death of the loved one prevented that from happening in person, the child can still have a "conversation" with the deceased in which these issues and feelings can be laid to rest. If the family's religious beliefs (discussed in the following section) are consistent with this perspective, the child may choose to have such a *mental conversation* with the deceased's soul or spirit. Other children will be more comfortable with the *reverse role-play* method, as described below. Another technique is having the child *write a letter to the deceased*, saying all the things the child wishes he/she could have said before the person died (Stubenbort et al., 2001). Whichever method is used, the goal is to have the child say the things he/she wishes had been said before the death and to imagine and verbally describe what the deceased would have wanted to say to the child, in order to resolve their unfinished business. Again, it may be helpful to have the child write a letter which he/she imagines the deceased would like to write to him/her. Care should be taken to not confuse the younger child into thinking the parent is alive somewhere (one usually sends letters to living people at distant locations). It may be helpful to put the letter in a balloon to send up into the sky (toward heaven) or to bury the letter in the ground for children who seem confused in this way (Worden, 1996).

The cognitive-processing techniques described earlier in this book can be used to process inaccurate or unhelpful thoughts about the deceased. Simply expressing these feelings may not resolve the child's ambivalence, particularly if the child experienced acts perpetrated by the deceased, such as child abuse or domestic violence. These traumatic experiences may not have been addressed during the trauma-focused sessions, which may have focused on the trauma that resulted in the deceased's death. Cognitive processing of the child's ambivalent feelings toward, and experiences with, the deceased may take several sessions at this point in therapy and should utilize the interventions described earlier in this book.

With regard to imagining a "healing" conversation to resolve problems with the deceased, some parents and therapists may feel uncomfortable encouraging the child to believe something about the deceased that would be "out of character," and may be concerned that this intervention would encourage unhealthy idealization of the deceased. The goal is not to alter the reality (or the child's perception) of what the deceased was like in life, but to allow the child to believe that despite these problems, the deceased loved the child and, at the end, would have wanted the best for the child. For example, the child whose father died of a drug overdose would be encouraged to believe that the father would want to say something like the following: "I was wrong for using drugs and I am sorry; I used drugs because of my own weakness and sickness, not because of anything about you; you were a great kid, and my biggest regret is that I missed out on being a better parent; you are strong and you will not end up like me; I love you and want you to be happy." Some parents may idealize the deceased themselves and have difficulty accepting that the child had negative feelings about the loved one (as discussed in the following section). It is important for the therapist to discuss this intervention with the parent/caretaker prior to introducing it in child sessions, not only to respect the parent's wishes in this regard, but also because the parent may have important insights about the deceased that can facilitate the therapist in this process. Finally, in the joint child–parent sessions, it is important for the parent to reinforce the child's belief that the deceased would have hoped to work out these issues before he/she died.

Another difficult aspect of grieving what was lost for some children might pertain to the fact that they were much closer to the deceased parent than to the surviving one; the child's ambivalent feelings might be toward the surviving parent, whom the child might even hold responsible in some way for the deceased parent's death. Assuming there is no basis in reality to the child's perception of the surviving parent's responsibility, this issue will need to be addressed with the parent and possibly in a family therapy context, which might provide a more in-depth focus.

GRIEVING THE LOSS AND ADDRESSING AMBIVALENT FEELINGS TOWARD THE DECEASED: FOR PARENTS

Grieving the Loss

The therapist should discuss with the parent what the child is expressing in therapy about his/her loss. It is expected that this discussion will prompt feelings of great sadness, just as it did for the child. Assuming that the parent had an ongoing relationship with the deceased, the parent will be grieving both the child's loss and his/her personal loss. The therapist should normalize these feelings and characterize them as feelings a good parent who loves his/her child would feel. It may be helpful to frame this point for the parent in the following manner:

> "Of course it fills you with sadness to hear about your child's sadness. It's hard for any loving parent to see her [his] child experience pain. But as a therapist, I am relieved that your child can experience this pain. So many children build a wall around their feelings and are afraid to feel anything at all in this situation. There is less pain, but these children will have trouble feeling other feelings, too—happiness, pride, enthusiasm, and other good feelings. Feeling sadness and pain is unfortunately a necessary step on the way

to healing, and I am grateful that your child is brave enough to let herself [himself] feel."

With regard to future losses implicit in the current loss, the parent may be able to suggest ways in which the child can optimally deal with these loss reminders in the future. The parent can try to anticipate some of these and recognize the importance of making these future events "special" for the child. For example, a parent who missed school plays or sporting events in the past because the deceased parent attended them might plan to attend these events regularly in the future in order to minimize the feelings of loss the child may experience. Inviting other friends or relatives to these events may be another way to keep the events special for the child even, in the absence of the deceased.

Addressing Ambivalent Feelings toward the Deceased

As noted in the child treatment section, the therapist should discuss with the parent any ambivalent feelings the child is expressing toward the deceased and help the parent understand the child's perspective in this regard. Some parents may be feeling similar ambivalence toward the deceased loved one, but any lack of consonance between the child's and parent's feelings needs to be addressed by the therapist. This may happen in either direction—that is, the parent may feel ambivalence whereas the child does not, or vice versa.

The therapist should help the parent understand that the child did not have the same relationship with the deceased that the parent had. Thus it is not surprising that they have different feelings about the deceased. The therapist should explore with the parent whether the child or parent is idealizing (or devaluing) the deceased. If either is occurring, cognitive-processing interventions may be helpful in restoring a more realistic view of the deceased. Since it is not clear that idealizing a deceased loved one is necessarily harmful, caution should be used in correcting children's or parents' overly positive views of deceased loved ones. The best approach may be to encourage the parent to accept the child's view of the deceased as being valid for the child and to focus on ways to help the child resolve "unfinished business" with the deceased regardless of whether or not the parent shares an identical view. One exception: If the deceased is the child's sibling, it may be difficult for the child if the parent is idealizing the sibling. When such idealization occurs, surviving children can begin to feel resentful of the parent's focus on the deceased sibling and the child may begin to feel as if they could never live up to their parent's idealized perception of that sibling. If this is the case, it may be helpful to share this concern with the parent and help the parent begin to talk about the deceased sibling in more realistic ways, particularly in the presence of the surviving children.

The parent should also receive support in resolving guilt and other personal "unfinished business" with the deceased. Few relationships are without ups and downs. It is therefore not surprising that many grieving parents had a less than perfect relationship with the deceased and are filled with guilt over things that they did or did not do with or for the deceased, sometimes over the course of many years prior to the trauma/ death. For example, a husband who had an extramarital affair, a wife who was uninterested in marital intimacy, a sister who stopped speaking to her sibling 5 years ago over an argument that was unresolved—all of these family members may feel overwhelmed with guilt and self-blame following the unanticipated death of the estranged family member. This may be magnified if the deceased died in a manner that made him/her into a hero (e.g., the New York City rescue workers in the 2001 terrorist attack). The therapist should encourage the parent to *reflect accurately on the totality of the deceased*, not just the manner in which he/she died. Although there may be legitimate regrets, there are usually some valid reasons for the parent's previous feelings and/or behavior toward the deceased; it is important for the parent not to lose sight of these feelings in the height of emotions following the traumatic loss. It is also likely that, in addition to the regretted action, the parent contributed many positive things to the relationship, which are being overlooked or mini- mized in the parent's current frame of mind. Finally, it may be helpful to remind parents that "hindsight is 20/20"; few people are blessed with the ability to see things with perfect clarity *while* they are happening. The parent should thus be encouraged to be a bit more generous in his/ her self-assessment. Use of the "best-friend" role play may be helpful in this regard.

The *"best-friend" role play* is a method by which the parent is encouraged to be more realistic and fair in his/her self-assessment. The therapist should instruct the parent to pretend that he/she is the parent's best friend. The therapist plays the role of the parent and expresses to the "best friend" the disparaging, guilt-ridden feelings the parent has been experiencing about him/herself. For example, the therapist might say to the "best friend": "I was the worst husband ever. I wouldn't let Jane take the job she wanted and now I feel terrible. She died unfulfilled because of my selfishness." The therapist then asks the "best friend" what he would say to that friend to make him feel better or see things more clearly. Through this role play, the parent often is more supportive of the "best friend" than he has been to him/herself. Once the parent has corrected the attributions in the role play (e.g., "You didn't do it out of selfishness; she told me that she didn't really want to go work, she just wanted the extra money. You were trying to keep her from getting too stressed out."), the therapist should encourage the parent to be his/her own best friend—that is, use these same methods of challenging his/her own distorted cognitions that he/she would use with a best friend (Deblinger & Heflin, 1996).

TROUBLESHOOTING

How do you deal with the situation where the child and parent are not in the same place in their resolution of ambivalent feelings toward the deceased, or in grieving what has been lost?

This is a fairly common scenario, and this is one reason why our treatment model encourages parents and children to be seen in separate individual sessions during the early stages of therapy. In some cases, the child is ready to talk openly about the deceased before the parent is comfortable doing so. We have found that many parents in this situation are able to move forward in their own grieving in order to help their children in therapy. For example, some parents have found themselves able to tolerate talking about difficult aspects of the deceased partner in order to help their child resolve conflicted feelings, when they could not have tolerated such a discussion for their own benefit. In other cases, the therapist may determine that it is better for the child and parent to proceed at their own individual paces. The therapist may keep the parent informed of the child's progress in this regard, while at the same time acknowledging and affirming that the parent is not at the same place emotionally and that this difference is normal and expected.

How about suicides? How do you balance the need to keep from stigmatizing the family versus not glorifying the act, etc.?

This is an important issue, especially among teens who need to hear the message that suicide is not glorified or rewarded in any way. The family should decide how to memorialize the deceased in a way that is meaningful to them, recognizing their ambivalent feelings about how he/she took his/her own life. The therapist can be helpful in this regard if the memorial service has not yet occurred when the family enters therapy.

What about when an infant has died?

There is a risk of parents and older children idealizing an infant to the detriment of the other children in the family. Because infants do not have a chance to grow up, we freeze them as "little angels" in our minds forever, but this is not fair to the older children in the family. The other children may collude in this as well, and it is up to the therapist and parents to prevent them from doing this.

Preserving Positive Memories
of the Deceased

PRESERVING POSITIVE MEMORIES FOR CHILDREN

Once the child has begun the process of grieving the deceased and what has been lost from the future, and has addressed unfinished business with the deceased, he/she may be able to focus on positive aspects of the relationship shared with the loved one. Recording and preserving these positive memories in a concrete manner is bound to produce some sad and painful feelings, but in many cases it also allows children to reexperience the joy and happiness they shared with the loved one. It is very important for children to realize that they still have the capacity—and permission—to be happy. Some children may want to make a memory book, memory box, memory collage, or other memorial (Worden, 1996), which consists of pictures, keepsakes (e.g., tickets to movies or sporting events, an old birthday gift, a favorite toy or book), photographs, hand-drawn pictures, and/or poems or other writings about the loved one. A few children have also put together videotapes or slide shows of their loved one. Some children have asked other family members and friends to contribute to their memory project, whereas others prefer to gather these memorabilia on their own. One child lamented that all of the family pictures had been lost in the house fire that killed her sibling. She decided to ask her sister's friends and various other family members to contribute their favorite pictures of her sister and their family to her book. Many of the sister's friends wrote stories for this book, which included loving and funny stories the sister had told her friends about the surviving sibling over the years. This was enormously meaningful to the child, who through this activity realized how important she had been to her sister. Recent advances in computer imaging make it even more convenient to reproduce borrowed or faded pictures. Children greatly enjoy this activity and often reconnect with other family members and friends in the process of making these books. Here are some ideas that children have written, drawn, or included in photographs in their memorials of the deceased:

- His/her favorite clothes
- Funniest habit
- Hobbies
- "The best time we ever had together"
- "Favorite things that he [she] gave me"
- "The nicest thing she [he] ever did for me"
- His/her favorite expressions/jokes

Children are encouraged to share these memorials with their parent/caretaker during the joint sessions and to continue adding to them after therapy is completed.

A therapeutic activity children may enjoy in this regard is writing the name of the deceased and filling in and illustrating a happy memory for each letter of the person's name. For example:

Doughnut lover
Acted in the senior class play
Very good brother
Ice cream expert
Did great imitation of Usher

Joked around with me
Only one who played Play Station with me
Nerd—always on computer
Egg McMuffins were his favorite
Space cadet—wore mismatched socks to church!

In some cases children may have difficulty remembering activities or events shared with the deceased, and the surviving parent may not have been present for these occasions. It may be helpful to ask others to provide memories in these situations (e.g., if the deceased parent attended the child's sporting events and the surviving parent did not, the child might ask the team coach or other team members what they remembered about the deceased parent's involvement). Younger children will typically have more difficulty recalling positive memories due to developmental considerations. Such children may benefit from looking at photographs of themselves with the deceased, writing stories about these photographs, drawing pictures of themselves with the deceased, and asking the surviving parent, older siblings, grandparents, etc., to help them recall happy times together with the deceased.

Many children will benefit from holding a *memorial service* for the deceased, even if there has already been a formal service. Such a service allows children to orchestrate their own special tribute to the deceased, which can be held in the therapy session, at home, at the cemetery, or wherever children choose, and should include the people, symbols, and words children wish to use to memorialize the loved one. The therapist should assist parents in supporting children to hold such services if they so desire.

For children who have lost multiple loved ones in mass disasters, there may be no surviving family members with whom to reminisce. This absence may leave the orphaned child with many challenges to memorializing: the potential loss of home, all physical reminders, and all family members who could assist the child in preserving past memories of the family that has been lost. In this situation, the presence of surviving community members or more distant relatives may be helpful, for although they may not have memories of the nuclear family's interactions, they may be able to assist the child in recreating a broader family history and thereby reestablishing a context in which the child can memorialize his/her loved ones and the family unit that has been lost. However, especially for younger children, such historical memories will be of less interest than what they have personally lost—the love, comfort, and support of the loved one who has died. Encouraging children to remember and memorialize these individuals through community commemorations may be helpful.

PRESERVING POSITIVE MEMORIES FOR PARENTS

The parent should also be encouraged to assist the child in recalling and preserving positive memories of the deceased. This may be difficult if the parent's own relationship with the deceased was problematic; in this situation, the therapist should help the parent understand why positive memories are important in order for the child's healing to proceed. As discussed in the child section above, the therapist should explain to the parent that allowing the child to attribute *benevolent intent* (i.e., he/she meant well and wanted good for the child) to the deceased is important, even if there were negative aspects of the deceased's treatment of the child. Benevolent intent does not erase any negative acts of omission or commission that occurred in the relationship between the child and parent. In fact, allowing the child to attribute benevolent intent to the deceased may enable the child to more accurately recognize the negative as well as positive aspects of the relationship (because the child feels less guilt about thinking "bad things" of the deceased).

The parent who had a good relationship with the deceased may be able to add many fond memories of the child's interactions with the deceased to the child's book, including things that occurred when the child was a baby or which the child has forgotten. The parent who is able to assist the child in this way (e.g., looking through old scrapbooks or photo albums with the child or discussing past happy events where the deceased was present) models the important message that it is good to have happy memories and OK to have happy as well as sad feelings about these memories. It also shows the child that the parent can emotionally tolerate talking about the deceased, and that doing so does not always have to cause sadness.

TROUBLESHOOTING

How do you address preserving positive memories in situations where the child and parent had very different relationships with the deceased? What if the parents were divorced, for example?

As noted above, preserving positive memories does not mean denying ambivalent feelings. However, parents need to recognize and accept that their feelings may be different from their children's, especially when the deceased is the child's parent. Therapists should use clinical judgment in determining what is in the child's best interest with regard to sharing the parent's personal experiences with and feelings regarding the deceased.

What if the child's positive memories of the deceased are not realistic? For example, what if the child's sibling or parent was abusive but the child's memories do not reflect this mistreatment?

This is a difficult clinical situation. Such a child (who could be expected to have ambivalent feelings) might be minimizing or denying such feelings for a number of reasons. These could include traumatic bonding, projective identification with the abuser, guilt related to the fact that the child may have wished something bad to happen to the abusive parent, and so on. Although the therapist may have explored these issues during the trauma-focused components of treatment, it is possible that such a child still has unambivalently positive memories of the deceased. That may be all right, as long as the child's attributions of the abuse and the death are not detrimental (e.g., self-blame) to his/her personal development. It is important to acknowledge, in very concrete terms, those things that the deceased may have done that were wrong so that the child recognizes and does not shoulder the blame for violence that may have taken place. It may be in the child's best interest to preserve unambivalent positive memories of the deceased parent even if these are not completely realistic. These memories may be open to examination as the child gains new levels of cognitive maturity.

What if the child's positive memories are realistic and the surviving parent's are overly idealized; for example, if the deceased was a sibling?

As noted earlier, this situation can create an impossible ideal for the surviving children to live up to—the "little angel" or "perfect child" image of the deceased, to which the bereaved parent clings as a memory of perfection that was never true when the child was alive. The therapist should explore with the parent what the reality of the deceased child's life was like, and also what this fantasy of perfection does to the surviving children.

Redefining the Relationship with the Deceased and Committing to Present Relationships

Throughout these grief-focused components, the therapist has encouraged the child to have mental "conversations" with the deceased, imagining what the loved one would say or would have wanted to say to the child if given the opportunity. Many children continue to have these mental interactions with their loved one long after the trauma/death. Although this behavior is normal, it is hoped that over time, the child will begin to *accept that the relationship with the loved one is not an interactive one in the present but rather a relationship of memory* (Wolfelt, 1991). Some children may feel guilty, as if they are betraying the loved one, when they gradually adjust to a present and future without him/her. But this is what the child *needs* to do in order to reinvest in present relationships.

REDEFINING THE RELATIONSHIP FOR CHILDREN

One intervention we have used in group and individual settings, is the use of a balloon drawing (Stubenbort et al., 2001): the child is given a drawing of two balloons, one floating away in the air, and one anchored on the ground. The floating balloon represents things the child has lost, whereas the anchored balloon symbolizes all that the child still possesses, including memories of the deceased. The child is asked to fill each balloon with words that describe what he/she has lost and what he/she still possesses. This activity allows the child to recognize that, although memories of the deceased remain, the interactive relationship is gone.

Recommitting to present relationships is an important step in enhancing the child's adaptive functioning. After the death of a loved one, it is normal to withdraw somewhat from one's usual activities and relationships for a time. Following a traumatic loss, the development of PTSD symptoms may contribute to the child's self-imposed isolation of him/herself to an extreme or unhealthy degree. This social isolation may prevent the child from accessing natural support systems, such as friends, teachers, the parents of friends, clergy and members of one's religious congregation, etc., who could be available to the child if the child were only available to them.

Even uncomplicated grief can interfere with the reciprocal nature of healthy relationships; the child is focused on the loss. In the case of traumatic grief, much of the child's psychic energy is consumed by intense reminders and attempts to avoid them. However, once the child has begun to accept the death and begins to turn back to the task of living, an important aspect of healing is that of reconnecting with other important individuals in his/her life. The energy that had been unavailable can now be reinvested in existing and new relationships (Rando, 1993; Worden, 1996). Cognitive coping (i.e., learned optimism) can help the child refocus on what he/she still possesses as opposed to what has been lost. The therapist should ask the child to create a list of significant people and then identify (for each person) positive qualities, characteristics, or ways in which the person contributes to the child's life. Younger children can be directed to draw pictures of significant people, and the therapist can record the positive aspects for the child.

Therapists must be aware of obstacles to this important task of reinvesting. In addition to feelings of betrayal, children may also be wary of strong attachments for fear of additional losses. It is helpful for children to understand how their desire to protect themselves from pain and loss also prevents them from experiencing companionship and love. This point can be illustrated to children visually by having them draw themselves behind a wall and their pain (sad face), hurt (broken heart), and other negative feelings outside the wall. Allow children to discuss how good it feels to be able to keep that pain away. After they have completed this part of the intervention, the therapist can demonstrate (by drawing) how love (heart, people hugging, etc.) and other positive feelings and experiences are also unable to get through the wall. This step could then lead to a discussion about choosing to let the wall down a lit-tle at a time to allow for the possibility of positive relationships.

Layne, Pynoos, et al. (2001) describes "auditioning" others for roles that the deceased used to fill in the child's life. For example, a girl whose father died asked her uncle to coach her in basketball, but this uncle would have been totally unsuitable to help her with her calculus homework, so she asked her mother to help her with this. When she wanted to buy her mother a special gift for Mother's Day, she consulted her grandmother. All of these roles previously would have been filled by her father, so this girl had to figure out the best person to help her in each situation. Although none of these people took her father's place, she was better able to commit herself to current relationships and live in the present.

REDEFINING THE RELATIONSHIP FOR PARENTS

The child may need the parent's "permission" to let go of the relation-ship with the deceased as an interactive one; that is, the child may fear that letting go would be disloyal to the deceased, and may need the par-ent to dispute this idea. Doing so may be difficult for the parent who has not yet negotiated this transition him/herself. The therapist should help the parent understand that until the child can let go of the deceased, he/she will not be able to reinvest in present relationships—and that includes the ability to feel close to the surviving parent.

The therapist should explain that the child's ability to refocus on present and future relationships is crucial not only to grief resolution, but to the child's overall development as well. Most parents will want to do whatever it takes to help their child; therefore, understanding the importance of this task will enable them to move beyond their own grief to "do what's right" for their children. The therapist should explain to the parent that one of the major differences between the parent's and child's recovery involves the child's developmental stage. Specifically, the child is still a "work in progress," whereas the adult is assumed to be a full-formed, full-functioning being. A crucial task of development con-cerns the formation of identity. As social beings, children's identity development hinges, to a large degree, on their relationships with others, particularly significant others such as parents. It is through interactions with these significant persons that children learn who they are. If a child's "interactions" with a person who is no longer living continue to be primary, that relationship is one of the past. That is not to say that the deceased is no longer an important part of the child's life or an important aspect of who he/she is. However, in order for the child to continue to develop, he/she must have interactions with significant others who are a part of the living world and who will live, change, and grow along with the child. These significant adults provide "anchors" for the child to the world of the present and future, rather than allowing him/her to become stuck in the past. Providing such an anchor for a child will (1) ensure that the child is able to incorporate the positive aspects of the deceased parent into his/her developing identity, (2) promote a loving relationship with the surviving parent, and (3) enhance the likelihood that the child will be able to form positive, healthy relationships in the future (i.e., friends, teachers, a future spouse). It is helpful to assist the parent in focusing on what he/she desires for the child's future. When asked, most parents will report that one of the things they most want for their child is to have a loving wife or husband. Helping the parent to focus on their child's future may circumvent some of the resistance to viewing the relationship with the deceased as one in the present.

Once the parent has accepted the importance of this task and worked through any resistance, at least as it applies to the child, the therapist can review specific ways in which the parent can encourage redefining the relationship and investing in present ones. For example, the parent should be instructed to "tune in" to the language he/she uses when talking about the deceased. Does he/she refer to the deceased in the present or past tense? The parent and others should be encouraged to use past tense whenever possible (e.g., "Daddy *worked* at the bakery" versus "Daddy *works* at the bakery"). The parent does not necessarily need to correct the child's language but should use his/her own language (i.e., past tense) as a powerful way of modeling that the family is moving into the present. Encouraging any steps toward maintaining or developing relationships is also important. Just as a parent uses praise to increase other positive behaviors, his/her praise of appropriate social behaviors can be effective as well. The parent should praise the child for wanting to spend time with grandparents or friends. Simply stating "That sounds like a fun thing to do" or "I'm glad you're doing that, I want you to have fun with your friend" helps to relieve any guilt or reluctance the child might be experiencing. Some children feel guilty about leaving the surviving parent, and may need to hear directly that the parent is OK spending some time alone. The parent can model this behavior for children by spending time with his/her own friends or other relatives. Afterward, it may be helpful for the parent to initiate a discussion about thoughts and feelings during the child's time spent with others.

CONCERNS ABOUT ABILITY
TO RAISE CHILDREN ALONE

This discussion relates to situations in which the deceased is one of the child's parents. Whereas some bereaved parents carried the primary responsibility for child-rearing activities prior to the trauma/death, others assume these responsibilities for the first time in the aftermath of the loss. In either case, the bereaved parent often feels overwhelmed with the idea that he/she is alone in making all the decisions about the child's health, education, financial future, etc., which in the past had been shared to a varying extent with the deceased parent. As the seriousness of this responsibility becomes clear, the parent may feel a variety of emotions: fear or anxiety about being able to make the right decisions, anger or resentment toward the deceased for leaving this burden on him/her, and/or sadness about not having the deceased parent to lean on, share decision making with, and share the joy of watching the child grow up together. These feelings may be complicated by the deceased parent's previous decisions (e.g., to not get life insurance or not save for college; to insist on the child attending private school, to which the child is now accustomed but for which the surviving parent will no longer be able to pay; discouraging the surviving parent from developing a career). Allowing the parent to openly express these feelings may assist in their resolution. Cognitive distortions and misinformation can also be challenged and corrected in this process. For example, the belief "I don't know how to pay the bills; my husband did all of that" can be addressed by pointing out that paying bills is mostly a matter of being organized, that the mother has been organizing many things in the household for years, and that she can learn to do this as well. As noted above, one of the therapist's most important interventions may be the provision of the parent with appropriate information about legal, financial, medical, and other assistance programs. Finally, the therapist can point out that the parent *is* raising the children alone at the moment, and doing it well despite great adversity.

TROUBLESHOOTING

What about parents who make children feel guilty about "moving on"? How can the therapist address that issue without seeming insensitive to the parent's pain?

One way to address this issue is to point out children's developmentally normal focus on the present moment, and how adaptive this focus can be in helping them cope with challenges such as grief. If the parent perceives this behavior as "insensitivity," the therapist can gently reframe the child's emotions and behavior as healthy adaptation. The therapist may then explore the parent's fears or concerns about the child reinvesting in present relationships (e.g., that the child will forget the deceased) and present evidence to reassure the parent in this regard (e.g., that the child still talks about the deceased in every therapy session). The therapist may also, if appropriate, explore the parent's feelings of guilt and fears of letting go of an interactive relationship with the deceased and recommitting to present relationships (e.g., "If I am able to move on and start dating, that means I never really loved him," or "I would be a superficial person if I moved on," or "If I'm ready to move on, then I don't really deserve the insurance money," or "My in-laws will hate me if I move on.").

How do you help grandparents or other relatives who are raising orphaned children?

When children have lost both parents, the new caretakers may have extra challenges in helping the children commit to these new primary relationships. The children have lost their only parents in traumatic circumstances, and they will naturally feel torn loyalties in recommitting to new caretakers. If the new caretakers are sensitive to these feelings and encourage children's loyalties and memories of the deceased parents, they may be able to ease the transition. Making overt statements that they know they cannot ever, and would never want to, replace the deceased parents may relieve some of these anxieties in the children.

How do you address the situation of a child who wants his/her parents to have a new baby to replace a sibling who died? Is this a good idea or not?

This decision will probably not be left up to the therapist! The parents need to make this decision based on their own desire to have another child, not the child's desire to have them replace a lost sibling. No new child should have the burden placed upon him/her of having to *replace* the lost child. The concept of reinvesting in new relationships suggests that this child would be better served by moving beyond the nuclear family to find other children with whom to be close, if the parents choose not to have another child. The therapist can work with such a child to explore alternative ways for him/her to develop satisfying relationships with peers.

Treatment Review and Closure

As the end of therapy approaches, the therapist should assess how the child and parent are progressing in treatment. If they are each showing improved adjustment, the therapist should suggest the possibility of having one or two more joint sessions toward the end of treatment. This possibility should be presented as an opportunity to share the child's completed trauma- and/or grief-related work and to acknowledge the gains both child and parent have made in treatment. It is important that these joint sessions be planned ahead of time so that the final treatment session can still be utilized for a therapy graduation celebration.

Preparation for the final joint sessions should use the same format as did the earlier joint trauma-focused sessions: that is, the 15-minute individual child and parent sessions preceding the joint sessions should consist of sharing the child's work and preparing for joint child and parent activities. The parent should also practice appropriate responses. Whatever activities the child and parent agree to share together—for example, reading the child's books, poems, or letters; sharing positive memories; conducting memorial services; offering mutual praise—some time should be spent planning for future loss and trauma reminders.

The final session should be spent, in part, discussing the joint-session experiences, including thoughts and feelings of the child and parent experienced during these interactions. Additionally, the child's and parent's progress in therapy should be reviewed and acknowledged by the therapist, with appropriate praise given to each. If the therapist believes that either needs ongoing therapy, this recommendation should be discussed and appropriate referrals and arrangements made prior to treatment termination.

This final phase of the child's therapy should emphasize an issue that is salient to both trauma and grief: finding meaning in life after trauma or loss. Jacobs (1999) believes that CTG includes an existential component characterized by the feeling that life is meaningless and empty, and that one will never be able to escape the void left by the death of the loved one. Children who have suffered trauma or loss may experience a combination of these features of emptiness and may need assistance in making meaning out of the traumatic experience. The type of meaning to which we refer could be likened to finding the "silver lining" in a negative situation. Doing so enables the person to integrate what was a traumatic experience into his/her existing identity and world view, to refocus on the positive, and to begin once again to be future, rather than past, oriented.

To assist the child in "making meaning," the therapist can ask a series of questions:

> "If you met another child who had suffered the same kind of trauma or loss that you did, what would you want to tell him [her] about what you have learned?"
> "What would you want this child to know that might help him [her]?"
> "If this child thought therapy would be too hard, what would you say to him [her]?"
> "What do you think about yourself now that you've gone through this?"

The answers to these questions should be used to develop a summary of the child's advice to others, which would reflect the child's experience of progressing through treatment and the process of recovery. One child, for example, wrote: "I would want to say, 'I know what you feel like, it hurts really bad. . . . You want to pretend it didn't happen, but you really can't. . . . You have to talk about it and then it will get better. I know that no one can take away the love my mom felt for me. I think she is proud of me for getting through this." In addition, answering these types of questions from a position of having been "through" something rather than being "in" it underscores to the child that he/she has moved beyond the traumatic event(s). Further, putting the child in a position of authority conveys a level of mastery and allows him/her to experience the rewards that come with the belief that he/she is helping another child. The child is thus contributing comfort to another child in a way that he/she imagines might have been helpful to him/her in the beginning of his/her grief or traumatic experience.

Here are some statements children have made about CTG treatment that convey what the experience has meant to them:

"You are not alone."
"I want other kids to know they will be OK."
"I learned the abuse wasn't my fault."
"You can be happy again."
"Your loved one is looking down on you from heaven."
"Even though the person is not here with you, you can carry him [her] in your heart."
"I found out how strong I am."
"I can still have fun."
"I found out who my true friends are."
"My dad and I got closer."
"It hurts at first but then I remember the good things."
"It's OK to remember."
"Talking about the death helps."

Another valuable way in which to assist children in making meaning is to identify a "corrective activity" for them to experience. Corrective activities are positive behaviors children can engage in that are somehow related to the trauma or loss. (Parents, however, should be consulted in advance regarding such activities to ensure that they are comfortable supporting their child's efforts.) For example, a child whose father died of a drug overdose may choose to speak to other students about the dangers of drug use. A child who experienced sexual abuse or exposure to domestic violence might want to contribute to an educational art exhibit about family violence. A child who lost a parent in the attack on the Word Trade Center may choose to visit the fire department to thank the firefighters for trying to rescue her parent (or may choose to write a letter to the firefighters or draw a picture for them). Again, these activities provide opportunities for mastery, the experience of helping others, and making meaning out of trauma or loss.

In a similar manner, parents can turn their most difficult experience into something positive by engaging in activities that help others to cope when faced with similar tragedies. An example of this type of activity is the USAir Flight 427 Support League, mentioned previously, which was established by surviving loved ones of victims of that airline crash, which occurred in 1994. This league has traveled around the United States to provide assistance and support to family members of other airline crash victims, and has had a major impact on how airlines address the needs of these survivors (Stubenbort et al., 2001).

Finally, the therapist should prepare for treatment termination by teaching the child the "three P's": *predict*, *plan*, and *permit*:

- *Predict* to the child that he/she will have times of sadness and grief throughout various points in life. These may be triggered by loss reminders (or trauma reminders).
- *Plan* for how to cope optimally with these reminders. This plan may include talking to a parent or other significant person, using a specific relaxation technique, visiting a memorial site, looking at a grief book, or any other activity that will bring the child comfort.
- *Permit* the child to have these feelings at any point in life, and have the child give permission to other family members to have and express these feelings without construing them as a sign of pathology. Parents also need to learn and practice the three P's and to reinforce them in their children.

One exercise that children have found helpful is creating a Circle of Life, a circular calendar with every month represented. (A sample Circle of Life is included in Appendix 1.) The child fills in each date that may serve as a trauma, loss, or change reminder in the coming years; for example, birthdays, holidays, graduations, first days of school, anniversary of the death or trauma, etc. The child also prepares for these dates by planning what he/she will do to comfort him/herself on that day. This is an activity that lends itself to sharing during the joint child–parent sessions.

As in any therapeutic relationship, termination and closure issues need to be addressed in a planned manner when utilizing the TF-CBT model. If this model is being provided in a highly structured manner (i.e., such that the treatment sessions are planned by the therapist and family to be limited to a specific number), the therapist may remind the family near the end of therapy that there are only two or three treatment sessions remaining, and that any outstanding issues should be addressed in that time frame. In clinical settings involving more flexibility regarding the number of treatment sessions, the therapist and family should discuss and plan for termination when the TF-CBT components have been addressed and adequately mastered, and when the child's and family's adaptive functioning indicates that treatment is no longer needed.

The therapist needs to be aware of, and sensitive to, the particular loss issues common to many traumatized children and how loss of a trusted therapist may resonate with these issues. Specifically, many traumatized children have sustained previous losses of loved ones (e.g., through violence, accidents, war, or through the conviction and imprisonment of a familial perpetrator of abuse). The subsequent loss of the therapist may bring to the fore abandonment or loss issues, and these should be addressed openly in the termination phase of therapy. It may be helpful to focus on the gains the child has made in therapy (such that he/she no longer needs to come to treatment every week but instead can spend this time on fun activities); on the increased availability, supportiveness, and efficacy of the parent, which has resulted from the family's hard work in therapy; and on the fact that the therapist is not leaving the child but rather the child is leaving the therapist (similar to graduating from one grade and being promoted into a new school). Finally, the therapist may choose to make him/herself available to the child in the future, should this option be clinically indicated. Indeed, this option may be particularly important for children and caregivers who anticipate potential trauma-related stressors in the future (e.g., court appearances). It is important to express both confidence in the child's abilities to manage such stressors on his/her own while also emphasizing that a return to therapy need not be seen as a failure but rather as a refresher course that can assist the child in getting through difficult and/or new developmental challenges.

Some children benefit from taking a memento of the therapist (e.g., a snapshot of the child and therapist together) or giving the therapist a snapshot of him/herself to keep. Assuring the child that the therapist will remember and continue to care about the child and family is also important. In summary, the TF-CBT model provides an important therapeutic relationship to the child and parent, and this relationship should be terminated in a planned and sensitive manner. For therapists desiring additional training or therapeutic resources related to the TF-CBT model, we have included links and other resource materials in Appendix 3.

TROUBLESHOOTING

How do you help children whose "meaning" about their traumatic experience is negative (e.g., "You can't count on anything in life")?

Additional cognitive processing might be warranted for such children who have overly pervasive or permanent negative cognitions in relation to their trauma or loss.

How do you help families when the parent's focus is on getting revenge or on the legal aspects of a case rather than on the child's therapy?

We have treated families where the parent's focus was on suing the airline or the murderer or the driver of the car that killed their loved one, or on the criminal trial of the sex offender, to the detriment of his/her involvement in the child's therapy. Because awards in civil cases sometimes depend on demonstrating damage, these parents may be inadvertently invested in keeping their children symptomatic or "sick" in order to prove to a jury how much damage has been done to their family as a result of their loved one's death. Needless to say, this stance does not contribute to a positive outcome in therapy; pointing this fact out to the parent may be helpful in refocusing attention on the child's current symptoms and need for treatment. In fact, it is important to emphasize to the parent that his/her potential influence on the child's recovery is much greater than the parent's ability to influence the offender's future and/or the legal outcome.

How do you help children who cannot tolerate their parent crying about the death or trauma?

Pointing out again the three P's—predicting the need and giving permission to grieve and planning how to cope optimally with these times—may be helpful to some children. Others may need their parent to reassure them that even though they are sad and crying, they are OK, they love the child and they just need a chance to let their feelings out. It may also be helpful for such children to hear that their presence gives the parent great happiness and comfort, because otherwise these children may wonder, "Am I not good enough to make up for your loss? Do I not make you happy? If I had been the child to die and the other child had lived, would you have been happy all the time?" Open discussion of these issues will go a long way to reassure children in this regard.

APPENDIX 1

HANDOUTS

DOMESTIC VIOLENCE INFORMATION SHEET
FOR PARENTS

WHAT IS DOMESTIC VIOLENCE?

Domestic violence is a pattern of control over the behavior, emotions, and choices of a partner. The methods of control can include physical abuse, sexual abuse, psychological abuse, financial abuse, social restrictions, and the destruction of property and/or family pets. Other terms that are often used when referring to domestic violence include, but are not limited to, *spouse abuse, intimate partner violence,* and *battering*. Regardless of the term used, domestic violence is a social problem where one's property, health, or life is endangered as a result of the intentional behavior of a partner. Current estimates are that in heterosexual relationships, domestic violence is most frequently committed by men against women. Domestic violence is as frequent in gay and lesbian relationships as in heterosexual ones. Domestic violence is also believed to be largely underreported.

WHAT ARE THE EFFECTS OF DOMESTIC VIOLENCE ON CHILDREN?

Being exposed to domestic violence affects children's emotional, developmental, and physical well-being. These children are more likely to be abused themselves, may be caught in harm's way during a violent episode and be inadvertently injured, may experience behavioral problems related to anger, aggression, and oppositional behaviors, and are more likely to experience depression and anxiety than other children. They also tend to spend less time with their friends, worry more about the safety of their friends, and are less likely to have a best friend. At school, children exposed to domestic violence may present with elevated rates of behavior problems, hyperactivity, social withdrawal, and learning difficulties.

Many of these children develop symptoms of posttraumatic stress disorder (PTSD) due to exposure to domestic violence. These symptoms include, but are not limited to, distressing memories and/or nightmares of the violence; efforts to avoid thoughts, feelings, or conversations that may remind

(continued)

them of the violence; diminished interest in activities that were once pleasurable; social isolation; difficulty falling or staying asleep; difficulty concentrating; and anger outbursts.

Children exposed to domestic violence are also at a higher risk of being exposed to other forms of abuse. It is currently estimated that 50% of perpetrators who abuse their spouses also abuse their children. These children have also been found to be at a higher risk of being emotionally abused and sexually abused than other children.

Exposure to domestic violence may also cause other long-term effects such as an increased risk of entering the juvenile justice system, attempting suicide, committing sexual assault crimes, and abusing drugs and alcohol. There is also an increased risk of becoming victims of abuse as adults and of developing distorted belief systems in regard to relationships, personal responsibility, violence and aggression, and sex-role expectations.

Every child responds to domestic violence exposure differently due to the influence of such characteristics as age, length of time the abuse has occurred, frequency and severity of the abuse, the child's relationship with the abuser, type of abuse, support system available to the child, and the child's overall resiliency and vulnerability.

HOW COMMON IS DOMESTIC VIOLENCE?

Domestic violence occurs across all races, religions, ethnicities, and economic groups. It is estimated that more than 1 million women are victims of domestic violence every year, with a high percentage of these assaults being witnessed by one or more children. In other words, more than 3 million American children are exposed to domestic violence each year.

WHAT ARE SOME COMMON BEHAVIORAL SYMPTOMS OF A CHILD WHO HAS BEEN EXPOSED TO DOMESTIC VIOLENCE?

- Bullying, physical aggressiveness, and insulting behavior toward peers.
- Withdrawal from peers and social contacts, and overall poor peer relationships.
- Difficulty separating, especially from the battered parent.
- Oppositional and defiant behaviors with authority figures, especially with the battered parent.

(continued)

- Increased verbal aggressiveness/talking back.
- Bed-wetting, daytime "accidents," "baby talk," or other regressive behaviors.
- Difficulty focusing and leaning while at school.
- Loss of appetite or changes in eating patterns.
- Failure to thrive in infants.
- Nightmares, insomnia, or other sleep problems.
- Increased violent behavior toward siblings and peers.
- Running away from home.
- Role reversal: taking on parental role.

WHAT ARE SOME BEHAVIORAL SYMPTOMS IN PRETEENS AND TEENAGERS WHO HAVE BEEN EXPOSED TO DOMESTIC VIOLENCE?

- Physically, verbally, or sexually abusing their dating partners.
- Being victimized physically, verbally, or sexually *by* their dating partners.
- Violence toward the battered parent/imitating words and behaviors of the abuser.
- Acting as the battered parent's "protector."
- Drug and/or alcohol abuse.
- Poor peer relationships and choices.

WHAT ARE SOME EMOTIONAL SYMPTOMS OF EXPOSURE TO DOMESTIC VIOLENCE?

- Increased nervousness, anxiety, and fear.
- Depressed mood and suicidal thoughts.
- Insecurity.
- Feeling responsible for protecting the battered parent and siblings.
- Excessive worry about the safety of others.
- Embarrassment (not wanting peers to be aware of family violence).
- Resentment toward the battered parent and siblings.

(continued)

- Fear of day-to-day arguments.
- Fantasies of standing up to, or hurting, the abuser.
- Desire to have the same power as the abuser.
- Confusion regarding "loyalty" to both the abusive and abused parent.

WHO PERPETRATES DOMESTIC VIOLENCE?

A perpetrator or "batterer" is a person who exercises a pattern of coercive control in a partner relationship, with one or more acts of intimidating physical violence, sexual assault, or threatening physical violence. This pattern may be manifested in the form of psychological control, economic control, sexual coercion, or primarily through physical violence. Although there are batterers in both sexes, most are male. Even though the batterer may be violent only toward his (or her) partner, he (or she) is also the person responsible for exposing the child to the violence. Battering is not due to impulse control problems, drinking problems, or anger management problems. It is a problem of intentional, repeated coercive controlling behavior that one partner exerts over the other in an intimate relationship. For this reason, anger management, Alcoholics Anonymous, or couple therapy are not the appropriate treatments to stop domestic violence.

HOW CAN I HELP MY CHILD?

- Tell him/her that abusive behavior is wrong.
- Reassure your child that none of the violent episodes were in any way his/her fault.
- Remind your child how much you love him/her.
- Develop a safety plan to prepare for crisis situations.
- Encourage your child to talk openly about his/her feelings.
- Prepare to get extra help for your child's schooling.
- Seek help from a mental health professional.

DOMESTIC VIOLENCE INFORMATION SHEET FOR CHILDREN

WHAT DOES DOMESTIC VIOLENCE MEAN?

Domestic violence means that one adult family member is hurting another family member. This "hurt" can occur when an adult pushes, shoves, hits, slaps, punches, or uses objects to hurt another family member. The hurting can also occur through name calling, not allowing someone to do what he/she wants, making a person do things that he/she doesn't want to, and by threatening to push, hit, slap, punch, or even kill the person. This can all seem very scary, but the most important thing to remember is that when adults fight, it's *never* the child's fault. Children can't stop the fighting between the adults in their home, no matter how good they are.

ARE THERE A LOT OF KIDS WHO SEE AND HEAR DOMESTIC VIOLENCE IN THEIR HOMES?

Yes. More than 3 million kids see this violence in their homes every year. This means that there are lots of children who see and hear adult family members hurting one another.

WHAT CAN KIDS DO TO HELP THEMSELVES WHEN THEY SEE OR HEAR THIS KIND OF VIOLENCE IN THEIR HOMES?

1. When there is no fighting, they can talk to their parents about how it feels when one parent hurts another.
2. Plan with their parents to have a "safe" house or place where they can go when their parents are fighting.
3. Come up with a safety plan with the battered parent in case of emergencies.
4. Talk to a grandparent, aunt or uncle, a grown-up friend, a friend's parents, or a family helper about how they feel when their parents fight.

(continued)

From Judith A. Cohen, Anthony P. Mannarino, and Esther Deblinger. Copyright 2006. Permission to photocopy this handout is granted to purchasers of this book for personal use only (see copyright page for details).

5. Draw pictures of what they are feeling.

6. Do things that make them happy, such as reading favorite books, playing board games or video games, watching TV shows, and talking to friends on the phone (or visiting them).

7. Remember that they are not the reason one parent is abusing the other.

WHAT CAN KIDS DO IF THEY ARE FEELING UNHAPPY OR SCARED, EVEN IF THEY NO LONGER LIVE WITH THE PERSON WHO WAS VIOLENT TO THEIR ABUSED PARENT?

1. Talk to the abused parent or other trusted adult about how it felt when they saw or heard the violence in their home.

2. Talk to the abused parent or other trusted adult about what it feels like now that things are different, even if the feelings are confusing.

3. Talk to a family helper about all of these confusing feelings.

4. Do things to help them feel happy, such as drawing, reading, coloring, playing board games, playing video games, watching TV, playing sports, and spending time with family and friends.

5. Remember that no matter what had happened between their parents, it was *not* their fault.

CHILD SEXUAL ABUSE INFORMATION SHEET FOR PARENTS

WHAT IS CHILD SEXUAL ABUSE?

Child sexual abuse is often defined as contacts or interactions between a child and an adult in which the child is used for the sexual gratification of the offender or another person. Sexual abuse may also be committed by a person under the age of 18 when the person is either significantly older than the child or is in a position of power or control over that child. Most often, sexual abuse involves some direct physical contact—e.g., sexualized touching and/or kissing; fondling, rubbing, and/or penetration of the vagina or anus with the fingers; oral sex; and simulated intercourse or penile penetration of the vagina or anus. Some sex offenders gratify themselves by exhibiting their genitals to a child or by observing or filming a child removing his or her own clothes.

Children are often engaged in these sexually abusive activities by playful coaxing (e.g., "This will be our special secret . . . ") or bribed with offers of money, candy, and favors. Sometimes they are bullied or threatened. On some less frequent occasions, physical force or violence may be used. It is important to remember that whether or not the child is actually "hurt," whether or not the child objects, and whether or not the child likes it, such sexual engagement by an adult or a coercive or older child is considered to be child sexual abuse.

WHAT ARE THE CONSEQUENCES WHEN CHILDREN EXPERIENCE SEXUAL ABUSE?

Children who have endured sexual abuse may experience a wide range of emotional and/or behavioral reactions to the abuse. The nature and severity of these difficulties may depend upon the age of the child, the identity of the offender, the circumstances of the abuse, and the family's reaction to the child's disclosure. Children may exhibit symptoms indicative of anxiety and distress, such as wetting the bed, withdrawn or acting-out behavior, nightmares, difficulty in school, and running away. These difficulties are

(continued)

similar to the problems exhibited by children who have experienced any kind of trauma. Children may also exhibit symptoms that are more specific to sexual abuse, such as repetitive sexual talk and play, age-inappropriate sexual behavior, and fears of specific situations or people that remind them of the abuse. Additionally, some children do not exhibit any apparent difficulties as a result of their traumatic experience.

Once the abuse has been disclosed and stopped, some children return to relatively normal behavior and emotions. The support and protection of the people close to them are very important in helping them get back to normal. However, some children have symptoms that persist long after the abuse itself has ended. In fact, a significant number of children who have experienced sexual abuse exhibit posttraumatic stress symptoms. That's why it's important for a child who has experienced sexual abuse to receive a psychological evaluation and, if necessary, treatment.

WHAT KIND OF TREATMENT IS AVAILABLE FOR CHILDREN WHO HAVE EXPERIENCED SEXUAL ABUSE?

Many therapy formats have been used to help children overcome the effects of sexual abuse. These include individual, family, and group therapy formats. The therapy techniques used have been derived from a wide range of psychological theories, including psychodynamic, behavioral, cognitive, insight-oriented, and structural and strategic theories of family therapy. There has been only limited research regarding the effectiveness of these varying approaches in assisting children to deal with the difficulties they experience as a result of sexual abuse. However, there is considerable research indicating that cognitive-behavioral therapy, applied in both individual and group settings, effectively decreases the problems experienced in the aftermath of sexual abuse.

Cognitive-behavioral interventions have been successful in helping children who have been sexually abused as well as their nonoffending caregivers. The cognitive-behavioral therapist may help nonoffending parents cope with their own thoughts and feelings about their children's abuse. At the same time, they teach parenting skills that help parents respond more effectively to their children's disclosures and abuse-related difficulties. Cognitive-behavioral interventions are individually tailored to target the particular child's difficulties and include educational, coping skills, and processing exercises. *Processing* exercises encourage children to confront memories, thoughts, and everyday reminders (e.g., bathrooms, sleeping alone, undress-

(continued)

ing, showering) of the abuse in a graduated fashion over time. Discussion, doll play, drawing, reading, writing, poetry, singing, etc., may be used in the process. By reducing the anxiety associated with abuse-related discussion, these therapy activities help children who have experienced sexual abuse to express their thoughts and feelings more openly, thereby enhancing their understanding and emotional processing of the abusive experience(s).

Finally, it is important for parents to know that the research in the field of child sexual abuse has repeatedly demonstrated that the most important factor influencing children's psychological adjustment following sexual abuse is the degree of support they receive from parents and other caregivers. With strong emotional support from caring adults and effective medical and mental health intervention, children who have experienced sexual abuse can look forward to healthy, satisfying, and fulfilling futures.

WHO IS SEXUALLY ABUSED?

Child sexual abuse cuts across all social classes and racial and religious groups. Both boys and girls are victimized, and it is not a very rare occurrence. Our best estimates suggest that, by the age of 18, one of every four females and one of seven males have been subjected to some form of contact sexual abuse.

WHO SEXUALLY ABUSES CHILDREN?

Although a small percentage of sex offenders are women, the majority are male. Sex offenders are generally *not* "dirty old men" or strangers lurking in alleys. They usually are not obviously mentally ill or retarded. In fact, sex offenders are often well known and trusted by the children they abuse. Offenders are often family members (e.g., cousin, uncle, parent, stepparent, grandparent) or individuals who are unrelated but well known to the child (e.g., a neighbor, coach, babysitter). There is no clear-cut description or profile of a sex offender, and there is no way to recognize a potential abuser. For this reason, it is often hard to believe that a trusted individual would be capable of sexually abusing children.

Some offenders have been sexually abused themselves as children. Others have suffered other forms of abuse and neglect in childhood. Some may be unable to function sexually with adult partners and may have many

(continued)

different encounters with children. Others are able to maintain sexual relationships with adults, but may turn to children for gratification during times of stress. A small percentage of offenders sexually abuse children while the offender is under the influence of drugs or alcohol.

WHY DOES SEXUAL ABUSE OCCUR?

Although the question as to why child sexual abuse occurs is frequently asked by children and their caretakers, there is no simple answer. *The main point to remember is that children and adolescents who have experienced sexual abuse and their nonoffending parents are not to blame.* The responsibility for sexual abuse rests squarely on the shoulders of the sex offender, regardless of the problems which may have contributed to his/her abusive behavior.

Our society is generally uncomfortable with sexuality and has made limited efforts to prevent child sexual abuse; these attitudes may also be responsible for keeping the problem hidden for so long. For this reason, it is essential that we communicate our concerns about child sexual abuse clearly and openly. As a society, we must become more aware of the seriousness and prevalence of the problem, and we must increase our present efforts to address this problem worldwide.

WHY DON'T CHILDREN TELL US WHAT'S HAPPENING?

Child sexual abuse is, by its very nature, secretive. It almost always occurs when a child is alone with an offender. In order for the sexual activity to continue, offenders rely on the children to keep the secret. There may be direct threats of physical harm to the children and/or to their pets, family members, etc., if they tell. Often children are led to believe that the abuse is their own fault and that they will be blamed, rejected, or disbelieved if they tell. They feel embarrassed, ashamed, and fearful about the abuse as well as the secrecy. In fact, many children who have experienced sexual abuse grow to adulthood without ever telling anyone because they fear rejection, punishment, or retaliation.

(continued)

WHEN SHOULD YOU SUSPECT CHILD SEXUAL ABUSE?

Because of the secretive nature and wide range of behavioral reactions of children, child sexual abuse is a difficult problem to detect. Children who have been sexually abused, however, are most often identified as a result of their own accidental or purposeful disclosures. Some children accidentally reveal their abuse by exhibiting adult-like sexual behaviors or by sharing sexual knowledge that is beyond their years. Some children may make a vague disclosure or tell a friend who then tells an adult. Parents should be aware of sudden changes in behavior: nightmares, withdrawal, and avoidance of particular persons, places, or things, unusual aggressiveness, jumpiness, and/or inappropriate sexual behavior. These behaviors may suggest the presence of a wide range of possible traumatic difficulties that need to be explored.

Children's reactions to the person who abuses them are quite varied. One cannot determine if sexual abuse is occurring by observing the child and alleged offender together. Some children are fearful and/or avoid their offenders; others talk very negatively about the offender but behave positively to him/her. Still others remain very attached and loving to an offending parent or caretaker. Whether they are positive, negative, or ambivalent, the child's feelings toward the offender should be accepted. Children need to know that none of their feelings is wrong.

Teaching your child personal safety skills and maintaining open lines of communication within the family may increase the likelihood that your child would disclose sexual abuse and/or other traumatic childhood experiences, if experienced.

HOW CAN YOU REDUCE A CHILD'S RISK OF SEXUAL VICTIMIZATION?

It is important to maintain open lines of communication with children, in general. Specifically, children should receive age-appropriate sex education as well as information about sexual abuse. Just as we teach our children about fire prevention, we also need to teach them about child sexual abuse. Children should be taught, in a matter-of-fact way, that their bodies belong to them and that they have the right to say "no" to a "not OK" touch. They need to be taught that they can tell an adult about any touching that makes them feel uncomfortable or that they think is a "not OK." In addition, children and adolescents can be taught how to make safe deci-

(continued)

sions about where they go and what they do when there is no parental or adult supervision.

It is important to remember, however, that it may be extremely difficult for a child or an adolescent to stop, or tell about, sexual abuse. Therefore, *a child or adolescent should never be blamed for not stopping the abuse from happening or for waiting a while before telling about it.* Many children never tell, and most children don't tell right away.

It is also important to remember that parents cannot watch and supervise their children all the time. Thus, *no matter what you do, you may be unable to ensure that your child is never sexually abused.* As a nonabusive parent you should not blame yourself if your child is sexually abused. Instead, it is most helpful to devote your energy to obtaining the needed services for your child.

HOW SHOULD YOU RESPOND IF YOU SUSPECT CHILD SEXUAL ABUSE?

It's natural for parents to feel quite distressed upon discovering that their child may have been sexually abused. However, the most important action to take as a parent is to *try to remain calm.* Children, including adolescents, are very sensitive to parental emotional reactions, and if they see or feel how upset or angry you are, they may be very frightened and "clam up." You want to convey to your child that it's good that he/she has told you. If you can't question your child calmly by yourself, it is better to wait for help from a professional. Be careful not to say anything that sounds like you blame him/her, and be sure to emphasize that the abuse is not his or her fault. Some children report that the sexual contact felt good. This does *not* mean that the child is, in any way, to blame or that the child should feel guilty for having enjoyed the sexual interaction and/or the offender's attention. Sometimes children who have been victimized may even initiate sexual behavior with other adults. However, it is *always* the *adult's responsibility* to set appropriate limits.

Don't encourage your child to "forget about it" and shut off the conversation. On the other hand, it's not helpful to push the child beyond what he/she is ready to say. Just be open to whatever your child can tell you and to any questions he/she may ask. Try to understand that the child may have mixed feelings about the offender and what has happened. Although you may feel like keeping your child at your side continually for protection, it's important that you not be overly restrictive and that you help your family

(continued)

218

return to as normal a routine as possible. It's also important not to be afraid to show your child your normal expressions of affection and physical closeness. Sometimes this is difficult, especially for nonabusive fathers. But you don't want to give the child the impression that your feelings about him/her have changed because of what has happened.

Children who may have been sexually abused should undergo a specialized physical examination that includes the genital area. Although children may feel hurt by sexual abuse, their bodies usually remain unchanged. Well-trained physicians can reassure children that their bodies are OK.

WHERE SHOULD YOU GO FOR HELP?

Anyone who suspects that a child has been sexually abused should contact the child protection agency in his/her state. Most states have a 24-hour toll-free number for this purpose. You may remain anonymous, but the caseworker will ask you important questions about the child, the possible offender, and the circumstances. The agency will most likely investigate the sexual abuse allegations and provide guidance and help to the child and family.

CHILD SEXUAL ABUSE INFORMATION SHEET FOR CHILDREN

WHAT IS CHILD SEXUAL ABUSE?

Child sexual abuse occurs when an adult or older child touches or rubs a child's private parts (penis, testicles, vagina, bottom, breasts), or when an adult or older child asks a child to touch or rub the other person's private parts. This kind of touching is **not OK.** The person who does this is called a sex offender. The offender might make the child do these things and be rough, or he/she might pretend it's a game or even give the child a reward to do it. The offender could be someone known to the child—a relative, a family friend, a teenager, or another child. Still, it's not OK even if the person tries to make it fun, and the child thinks it's fun.

WHO IS SEXUALLY ABUSED?

Sexual abuse happens to a lot of children. It can happen to boys and girls of all ages, religions, and races. Some children who have been sexually abused are rich, some are poor, and they are all from different neighborhoods. By the age of 18, one of every four girls and one of seven boys may have experienced sexual abuse.

WHO SEXUALLY ABUSES CHILDREN?

Some people sexually abuse children, but many more people only touch children with *not* OK touches. Most sex offenders are men, though some are women. Children cannot tell by the way these people look, dress, or act that they are offenders. Most of the time, the offender is not a stranger but someone whom the child knows very well. The offender could be a family member (such as a cousin, uncle, parent, or grandparent) or someone who is well known to the child (such as a coach, babysitter, or neighbor).

(continued)

WHY DON'T CHILDREN TELL?

Sometimes the offender tells the child to keep the not OK touching a secret. The offender may use tricks to keep the child from telling. The person may say that it's the child's fault or that the child or his/her family will get hurt if the child tells. These are all tricks. Sometimes children just keep it a secret because they feel ashamed, embarrassed, or scared. For those reasons, many children don't tell about sexual abuse or they take a little while to gain the courage to tell. It helps the children to keep telling adults until they find an adult who will help them to stop the sexual abuse.

WHY DOES SEXUAL ABUSE HAPPEN?

There are lots of different reasons, just like there are lots of different offenders. But it's very hard to know the reason why it happens to any child. We do know this much: No child is responsible for what an adult does.

HOW CAN YOU TELL THAT A CHILD HAS BEEN SEXUALLY ABUSED?

You can't tell by looking at a child that he/she has been sexually abused. Sometimes you can tell by the way the child is acting that something is bothering him/her, but you don't know what it is. That is why it is so important for children to tell somebody when they experience a not OK or confusing touch.

HOW DO CHILDREN FEEL WHEN THEY HAVE BEEN SEXUALLY ABUSED?

Children may have all kinds of feelings in response to sexual abuse. The sexual touching may feel good to some children, and they may still like the person who did it. But some children have other feelings; they are very angry at the person who did the abuse or are scared of him/her. Other children might feel guilty about what happened. Any of these feelings is OK. Sometimes when people have these feelings, the feelings affect the way they behave. A child who is afraid may not want to sleep alone or be left alone. Sometimes children get into more arguments, and sometimes they

(continued)

221

may just feel sad and want to be alone. Some children feel upset for a long time after the abuse has ended, but they often feel better with the help of counseling. If children are having a hard time with these feelings, talking with a counselor or a parent can help them feel better.

HOW CAN CHILDREN RESPOND TO CHILD SEXUAL ABUSE?

All children need to know that their body belongs to them. If you feel uncomfortable in the way you are being touched, you can tell the person "NO!" Saying "NO!" can sometimes be hard to do, especially if you're scared, shy, or embarrassed. But the next thing you can do is "GO"—get away from that person. And the next and most important thing to do is "TELL"—although this can also be hard to do, it is important to tell an adult (such as a parent, other family member, or a teacher) about what happened. It is important to keep telling until someone listens and helps. Remember the steps: NO–GO–TELL!

It's great to talk to a counselor or a parent. It helps to talk about sexual abuse, even though it can be hard. Talking, writing, and even singing and drawing can help children who have been sexually abused feel better after a while.

It's important to tell adults about child sexual abuse so that they can get help. There is a special agency in every state that is available to help children who have experienced abuse.

RELAXATION HANDOUT:
HOW STRESS AND PTSD AFFECT OUR BODIES

Stress affects us by stimulating the production of chemicals in different parts of our brains and bodies. When stress becomes chronic, as in PTSD, these changes are more difficult to reverse.

IN THE BRAIN

The *hypothalamus* produces a chemical called CRF, which stimulates the *pituitary gland*. The pituitary then releases a chemical called ACTH, which circulates throughout the rest of the body.

The *amygdala*, which is responsible for assigning emotional meaning to the things we hear, see, smell, and feel, starts giving more emotional meaning to things that would not ordinarily have so much meaning. For example, things that we usually don't see as being scary are now labeled *scary* by the amygdala.

The *prefrontal cortex* is a part of the brain that is responsible for extinguishing learned fear responses. In PTSD, the prefrontal cortex is not as active as usual, so these previously learned fear responses are not extinguished. This makes it harder for us to stop being afraid of things that scared us in the past, even when they are no longer happening.

Finally, in the brain, there is increased production and activity of the neurotransmitter *norepinephrine* (also called *noradrenaline*), which leads to an increased presence of *epinephrine* or *adrenaline* in the rest of the body.

IN THE REST OF THE BODY

ACTH from the pituitary gland acts on the *adrenal glands* (near the kidneys) to increase the production of *cortisol*. Increased levels of cortisol contribute to higher levels of epinephrine in the rest of the body. These higher levels lead to the following effects:

(continued)

- Increased heart rate
- Pounding heart
- Shortness of breath
- Sweating
- Weakness, dizziness
- Muscle tension
- Stomach upset
- Headaches
- Skin rashes
- Fight, flight, or freeze response

The good news is that all of these effects can be reduced through the use of relaxation.

AFFECTIVE MODULATION HANDOUT: WAYS TO FEEL BETTER RIGHT NOW

1. Stop whatever you are doing, close your eyes, and take 10 slow, deep breaths.

2. Visualize your "safe place."

3. Go to a quiet room and read a good book.

4. Listen to your favorite music.

5. Pray, meditate, or focus on your special relaxation phrase.

6. Listen to, watch, or read something funny.

7. Go outside and take a walk in a safe area.

8. Run in place for 5 minutes.

9. Call a friend.

10. Talk to a parent or other adult who understands and listens.

11. Write in your journal.

12. Volunteer.

13. Sing out loud.

14. Dance.

15. Tell yourself that things will get better.

16. Take a warm bath.

17. Make something with your hands—knit, sew, crochet, woodwork, paint, etc.

18. Tell yourself five good things about yourself.

19. Talk about your feelings.

20. Tell someone you love him/her.

21. Play with your pet.

22. Do something to help someone else.

PRACTICING THE COGNITIVE TRIANGLE DURING THE WEEK

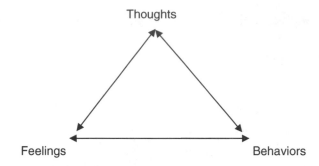

During the coming week, whenever you feel upset about something, write down the situation and how it makes you feel. Then "track back" to what your thought was about the situation that made you think that way. Ask yourself whether that thought is (1) accurate and (2) helpful. Come up with alternative thoughts in this situation and write down how they make you feel and whether they are accurate and helpful. To identify new, more helpful thoughts, think about what you would say to a good friend in a similar situation if he/she shared the distressing thought(s).

Situation: _____

Thought: _____

Feeling: _____

Behavior: _____

New thought: _____

New feeling: _____

New behavior: _____

(continued)

Situation: _____

Thought: _____

Feeling: _____

Behavior: _____

New thought: _____

New feeling: _____

New behavior: _____

Situation: _____

Thought: _____

Feeling: _____

Behavior: _____

New thought: _____

New feeling: _____

New behavior: _____

Situation: _____

Thought: _____

Feeling: _____

Behavior: _____

New thought: _____

New feeling: _____

New behavior: _____

THE CIRCLE OF LIFE

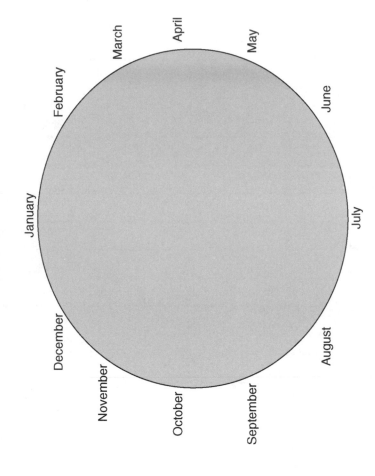

January
February
March
April
May
June
July
August
September
October
November
December

APPENDIX 2

RESOURCES

BOOKS FOR CHILDREN AND TEENS

Aboff, M. (2003). *Uncle Willy's tickles: A child's right to say no* (2nd ed.). Washington, DC: Magination Press.

Agee, J. (1957). *A death in the family*. New York: Bantam.

Aliki, (1979). *The two of them*. New York: Greenwillow Books.

Bean, B., & Bennett, S. (1993). *The me nobody knows: A guide for teen survivors*. New York: Lexington Books.

Buscaglia, L. (1982). *The fall of Freddie the leaf: A story of life for all ages*. Thorofare, NJ: Slack.

Cain, B. S. (2001). *Double-dip feelings: Stories to help children understand emotions*. Washington, DC: Magination Press.

Canfield, J., Hansen, M. V., & Kirberger, K. (Eds.). (1997). *Chicken soup for the teenage soul: 101 stories of life, love and learning*. Deerfield Beach, FL: Health Communications.

Curtis, J. L. (1998). *Today I feel silly and other moods that make my day*. New York: HaperCollins.

Deaton, W., & Johnson, K. (2002). *No more hurt: A growth and recovery workbook*. Alameda, CA: Hunter House.

de Paola, T. A. (1973). *Nana upstairs and Nana downstairs*. New York: Putnam.

Ditta-Donahue, G. (2003). *Josh's smiley faces: A story about anger*. Washington, DC: Magination Press.

Freeman, L. (1984). *It's my body: A book to teach young children how to resist uncomfortable touch*. Seattle: Parenting Press.

Gilgannon, D. (2000). *The hyena who lost her laugh: A story about changing your negative thinking*. Plainview, NY: Childswork/Childsplay.

Girard, L. W. (1984). *My body is private*. Morton Grove, IL: Albert Whitman.

Gray, A. (1999). (Ed.). *Stories for a teen's heart*. Sisters, OR: Multnomah.

Grollman, E. (1993). *Straight talk about death for teenagers: How to cope with losing someone you love.* Boston: Beacon Press.

Gunther, J. (1949). *Death be not proud: A memoir.* New York: Harper.

Harris, R. H. (2001). *Goodbye mousie.* New York: Margaret K. McElderry Books.

Harris, R. H., & Emberley, M. (1994). *It's perfectly normal: Changing bodies, growing up, sex and sexual health.* Cambridge, MA: Candlewick Press.

Harris, R. H., & Emberley, M. (1994). *It's so amazing: A book about eggs, sperm, birth, babies and families.* Cambridge, MA: Candlewick Press.

Hindman, J. (1983). *A very touching book . . . for little people and for big people.* Baker City, OR: Alexandria.

Holmes, M. M. (2000). *A terrible thing happened: A story for children who have witnessed violence or trauma.* Washington, DC: Magination.

Jessie (Sandra Hewitt). (1991). *Please tell!: A child's story about sexual abuse.* Minneapolis, MN: Hazelden Foundation.

Johnson, K. (1986). *The trouble with secrets.* Seattle: Parenting Press.

Kehoe, P. (1997). *Something happened and I'm scared to tell: A book for young victims of abuse.* Seattle: Parenting Press.

Kremnetz, J. (1988). *How it feels when a parent dies.* New York: Knopf.

Loiselle, M., & Wright, L. B. (1997). *Shining through: Pulling it together after sexual abuse.* (2nd ed.). Brandon, VT: Safe Society Press.

Madaras, L., & Madaras, A. (2000). *My body, my self for girls.* (2nd ed.). New York: Newmarket Press.

Mayle, P. (1975). *Where did I come from?: The facts of life without any nonsense and with illustrations.* New York: Kensington.

Mellonie, B., & Ingen, R. (1983). *Lifetimes: A beautiful way to explain death to children.* New York: Bantam.

Munson, L., & Riskin, K. (1995). *In their own words: A sexual abuse workbook for teenage girls.* Washington, DC: Child Welfare League.

Nass, M. S. (2000). *The lion who lost his roar: A story about facing your fears.* Plainview, NY: Childswork/Childsplay.

O'Toole, D. (1998). *Aarvy aardvark finds hope: A read aloud story for people of all ages about loving and losing, friendship and loss.* Burnsville, NC: Celo Press.

Paterson, K. (1977). *Bridge to Terabithia.* New York: Crowell.

Porterfield, K. M. (1996). *Straight talk about post-traumatic stress disorder: Coping with the aftermath of trauma.* New York: Facts on File.

Romain, T. (1999). *What on earth do you do when someone dies?* Minneapolis: Free Spirit.

Sanford, D. (1986). *I can't talk about it: A child's book about sexual abuse.* Sisters, OR: Gold'n Honey Books.

Sanford, D. (1993). *Something must be wrong with me: A boy's book about sexual abuse.* Sisters, OR: Quetar.

Smith, D. B. (1973). *A taste of blackberries.* New York: Crowell.

Sobel, M. (2000). *The penguin who lost her cool: A story about controlling your anger.* Plainview, NY: Childswork/Childsplay.

Sosland, M. (2005). *The can do duck: A story about believing in yourself.* Available from Can Do Duck Publishing, P. O. Box 1045, Voorhees, NJ, 08043; www.thecandoduck.com

Spelman, C. (1997). *Your body belongs to you.* Morton Grove, IL: Albert Whitman.

Stauffer, L., & Deblinger, E. (2003). *Let's talk about taking care of you!: An educational book about body safety.* Available from Hope for Families, Inc., P.O. Box 238, Hatfield, PA 19440; www.hope4families.com

Thomas, P. (2001). *I miss you: A first look at death.* Hauppauge, NY: Barrons.

Varley, S. (1984). *Badger's parting gifts.* New York: Lothrop.

Viorst, J. (1971). *The tenth good thing about Barney.* New York: Atheneum.

Wachter, O. (2002). *No more secrets for me* (rev. ed.). Boston: Little, Brown.

Weiner, M. B., & Neimark, J. (1994). *I want your moo: A story for children about self-esteem.* Washington, DC: Magination Press.

White, E. B. (1952). *Charlotte's web.* New York: Harper.

Wilgocki, J., & Wright, M. K. (2002). *Maybe days: A book for children in foster care.* Washington, DC: Magination Press.

Wright, L. B., & Loiselle, M. (1997). *Back on track: Boys dealing with sexual abuse.* Brandon, VT: Safe Society Press.

BOOKS FOR PARENTS

Clark, L. (1996). *SOS! Help for parents: A practical guide for handling common everyday behavior problems.* Bowling Green, KY: Parents Press.

Johnson, T. C. (2004). *Understanding children's sexual behaviors: A guidebook for professionals and caregivers.* Available from Toni Cavanaugh Johnson, 1101 Fremont Avenue, Suite 101, South Pasadena, CA 91030; www.tcavjohn.com

Patterson, G., & Forgatch, M. S. (2005). *Parents and adolescents living together, Part I: The basics.* Champaign, IL: Research Press.

Whitham, C. (1991). *Win the whining war and other skirmishes: A family peace plan.* Glendale, CA: Perspective.

PROFESSIONAL REFERENCES
ON CHILDHOOD BEREAVEMENT

Baker, J. E., Sedney, M. A., & Gross, E. (1996). Psychological tasks for bereaved children. *American Journal of Orthopsychiatry, 62*(1), 105–116.

Bowlby, J. (1973). *Attachment and loss: Vol 2. Separation: Anxiety and anger.* New York: Basic Books.

Christ, G. H. (2000). *Healing children's grief: Surviving a parent's death from cancer.* New York: Oxford University Press.

Dyregrov, A. (1991). *Grief in children: A handbook for adults.* London: Jessica Kingsley.

Emswiler, M. A., & Emswiler, J. P. (2000). *Guiding your child through grief.* New York: Guilford Press.

Fitzgerald, H. (1998). *Grief at school: A manual for school personnel.* Washington, DC: American Hospice Foundation. [Available from the American Hospice Foundation, 2120 L Street NW, Suite 200, Washington, DC 20037, www.americanhospice.org]

Geis, H. K., Whittlesey, S. W., McDonald, N. B., Smith, K. L., & Pfefferbaum, B. (1998). Bereavement and loss in childhood. *Child and Adolescent Psychiatric Clinics of North America, 7*(1), 73–85.

Grollman, E. A. (1995). *Bereaved children and teens: A support guide for parents and professionals.* Boston: Beacon Press.

Oltjenbruns, K. A. (2001). Developmental context of childhood grief. In M. S. Stroebe, R. O. Hansson, W. Stroeb, & H. Schut (Eds.), *Handbook of bereavement research: Consequences, coping, and care* (pp. 169–197). Washington, DC: American Psychological Association.

Rando, T. (1991). *How to go on living when someone you love dies.* New York: Bantam.

Smith, S. (1999). *The forgotten mourners: Guidelines for working with bereaved children* (2nd ed.). Philadelphia, PA: Jessica Kingsley.

Webb, N. B. (2002). *Helping bereaved children: A handbook for practitioners* (2nd ed.). New York: Guilford Press.

Wolfelt, A. D. (1996) *Healing the bereaved child: Grief gardening, growing through grief and other touchstones for caregivers.* Fort Collins, CO: Companion Press.

Worden, J. W. (1991). *Grief counseling and grief therapy: A handbook for the mental health professional* (2nd ed.). New York: Springer.

PROFESSIONAL REFERENCES ON CHILDHOOD TRAUMA AND TRAUMATIC GRIEF

Andrews, B. (1998). Shame and childhood abuse. In P. Gilbert & B. Andrews (Eds.), *Interpersonal behavior, psychopathology, and culture* (pp. 176–190). New York: Oxford University Press.

Andrews, B., Berwin, C. R., Rose, S., & Kirk, M. (2000). Predicting PTSD symptoms in victims of violent crime: The role of shame, anger, and childhood abuse. *Journal of Abnormal Psychology, 109,* 69–73.

Berliner, L., & Saunders, B. E. (1996). Treating fear and anxiety in sexually abused children: Results of a controlled 2 year study. *Child Maltreatment, 1,* 294–309.

Black, D. (1998). Working with the effects of traumatic bereavement by uxoricide (spouse killing) on young children's attachment behavior. *International Journal of Psychiatry in Clinical Practice, 2*(4), 245–249.

Brown, E. J., Pearlman, M. Y., & Goodman, R. F. (2004). Facing fears and sadness: Cognitive behavioral therapy for childhood traumatic grief. *Harvard Review of Psychiatry, 12*(4), 187–198.

Burgess, A. (1975). Family reaction to homicide. *American Journal of Orthopsychiatry, 45*(3), 391–398.

Cohen, B., Barnes, M.-M., & Rankin, A. (1995). *Managing traumatic stress though art*. Towson, MD: Sidran Press.

Cohen, J. A., Berliner, L., & Mannarino, A. P. (2000). Treatment of traumatized children: A review and synthesis. *Journal of Trauma, Violence and Abuse, 1*(1), 29–46.

Cohen, J. A., Deblinger, E., Mannarino, A. P., & De Arellano, M. A. (2001). The importance of culture in treating abused and neglected children: An empirical review. *Child Maltreatment, 6*(2), 148–157.

Cohen, J. A., Deblinger, E., Mannarino, A. P., & Steer R. A. (2004). A multisite, randomized controlled trial for children with sexual-abuse related PTSD symptoms. *Journal of the American Academy of Child and Adolescent Psychiatry, 43*, 393–402.

Cohen, J. A., & Mannarino, A. P. (1996a). A treatment outcome study for sexually abused preschool children: Initial findings. *Journal of the American Academy of Child and Adolescent Psychiatry, 35*(1), 42–50.

Cohen, J. A., & Mannarino, A. P. (1996b). Factors that mediate treatment outcome in sexually abused preschool children. *Journal of the American Academy of Child and Adolescent Psychiatry, 35*(10), 1402–1410.

Cohen, J. A., & Mannarino, A. P. (1997). A treatment study of sexually abused preschool children: Outcome during one year follow-up. *Journal of the American Academy of Child and Adolescent Psychiatry, 36*(9), 1228–1235.

Cohen, J. A., & Mannarino, A. P. (1998a). Interventions for sexually abused children: Initial treatment findings. *Child Maltreatment, 3*(1), 17–26.

Cohen, J. A., & Mannarino, A. P. (1998b). Factors that mediate treatment outcome of sexually abused preschool children: Six and 12-month follow-ups. *Journal of the American Academy of Child and Adolescent Psychiatry, 37*(1), 44–51.

Cohen, J. A., & Mannarino, A. P. (2004). Treatment of childhood traumatic grief. *Journal of Clinical Child and Adolescent Psychology, 33*(4), 820–832.

Cohen, J. A., Mannarino, A. P., Greenberg, T., Padlo, S., & Shipley, C. (2002). Childhood traumatic grief: Concepts and controversies. *Trauma Violence and Abuse, 3*(4), 307–327.

Cohen, J. A., Mannarino, A. P., & Knudsen, K. (2004). Treating childhood traumatic grief: A pilot study. *Journal of the American Academy of Child and Adolescent Psychiatry, 43*(10), 1225–1233.

De Arellano, M. A., Waldrop, A. E., Deblinger, E., Cohen, J. A., & Danielson, C. (2005). Community outreach program for child victims of traumatic events: A community-based project for underserved populations. *Behavior Modification, 29*(1), 130–155.

De Bellis, M. D., Keshavan, M. S., Clark, D. B., Casey, B. J., Giedd, J. N., Boring, A. M., et al. (1999). Developmental traumatology: Part II. Brain development. *Biological Psychiatry, 45*, 1271–1284.

Deblinger, E., & Heflin, A. H. (1996). *Treating sexually abused children and their nonoffending parents: A cognitive behavioral approach*. Thousand Oaks, CA: Sage.

Deblinger, E., Lippmann, J., & Steer, R. (1996). Sexually abused children suffering posttraumatic stress symptoms: Initial treatment outcome findings. *Child Maltreatment, 1*(4), 310–321.

Deblinger, E., McLeer, S. V., Atkins, M., Ralphe, D., & Foa, E. (1989). Post-traumatic stress in sexually abused, physically abused and nonabused children. *Child Abuse and Neglect, 13,* 403–408.

Deblinger, E., & Runyon, M. K. (2005). Understanding and treating feelings of shame in children who have experienced maltreatment. *Child Maltreatment, 10,* 364–376.

Deblinger, E., Stauffer, L. B., & Steer, R. (2001). Comparative efficacies of supportive and cognitive-behavioral group therapies for young children who have been sexually abused and their non-offending mothers. *Child Maltreatment, 6,* 332–343.

Deblinger, E., Steer, R., & Lippmann, J. (1999a). Maternal factors associated with sexually abused children's psychosocial adjustment. *Child Maltreatment, 4,* 13–20.

Deblinger, E., Steer, R. A., & Lippmann, J. (1999b). Two year follow-up study of cognitive behavioral therapy for sexually abused children suffering posttraumatic stress symptoms. *Child Abuse and Neglect, 23*(12), 1371–1378.

Deblinger, E., Taub, B., Maedel, A.B., Lippmann, J., & Stauffer, L. (1997). Psychosocial factors predicting parent reported symptomatology in sexually abused children. *Journal of Child Sexual Abuse, 6,* 35–49.

Eth, S., & Pynoos (1985). Interaction of trauma and grief in children. In S. Eth & R. Pynoos (Eds.), *Post-traumatic stress disorder in children* (pp. 171–183). Washington DC: American Psychiatric Press.

Felitti, V. J., Anda, R. F., Nordenberg, D., Williamson, D. F., Spitz, A. M., Edwards, V., et al. (1998). Relationship of childhood abuse and household dysfunction to many of the leading causes of death in adults: The Adverse Childhood Experiences (ACE) study. *American Journal of Preventive Medicine, 14*(4), 245–258.

Feiring, C., Taska, L. S., & Chen, K. (2002a). Trying to understand why horrible things happen: Attribution, shame, and symptom development following sexual abuse. *Child Maltreatment, 7,* 26–41.

Feiring, C., Taska, L., & Lewis, M. (2002b). Adjustment following sexual abuse discovery: The role of shame and attributional style. *Developmental Psychology, 38,* 79–92.

Foa, E. B., Johnson, K. M., Feeny, N. C., & Treadwell, K. H. (2001). The Child PTSD Symptom Scale: A preliminary examination of its psychometric properties. *Journal of Clinical Child Psychology, 30*(3), 376–384.

Foa, E. B., Zoellner, L. A., Feeny, N.C., Hembree, E. A., & Alvarez-Conrad, J. (2002). Does imaginal exposure exacerbate PTSD symptoms? *Journal of Consulting and Clinical Psychology, 70*(4), 1022–1028.

Follette, V. M., & Ruzek, J. I. (2006). *Cognitive-behavioral therapies for trauma* (2nd ed.). New York: Guilford Press.

Goldman, L. (2001). *Breaking the silence: A guide to helping children with complicated grief: Suicide, homicide, AIDS, violence and abuse.* Bristol, PA: Taylor & Francis.

Green, B. (1997). *Traumatic loss: Conceptual issues and new research findings.* Keynote address presented at the Fifth International Conference on Grief and Bereavement in Contemporary Society and the Nineteenth Annual Conference of the Association for Death Education and Counseling, Washington, DC.

Jacobs, S. (1999). *Traumatic grief: Diagnosis, treatment, and prevention.* Philadelphia: Brunner/Mazel.

Johnson, T. C. (1995). *Treatment exercises for child abuse victims and children with sexual behavior problems*; (2004). *Helping children with sexual behavior problems*; (2004). *Understanding your child's sexual behavior.* Available from Toni Cavanaugh Johnson, 1101 Fremont Avenue, Suite 101, South Pasadena, CA 91030.

Kehoe, P. (1988). *Helping abused children: A book for those who work with sexually abused children.* Seattle: Parenting Press.

King, N. J., Tonge, B. J., Mullen, P., Myerson, N., Heyne, D., Rollings, S., et al. (2000). Treating sexually abused children with posttraumatic stress symptoms: A randomized clinical trial. *Journal of the American Academy of Child and Adolescent Psychiatry, 39*(11),1347–1355.

Layne, C. M., Pynoos, R. S., & Cardenas, J. (2001). Wounded adolescence: School-based group psychotherapy for adolescents who have sustained or witnessed violent injury. In M. Shafii & S. Shafii (Eds.), *School violence: Contributing factors, management, prevention* (pp. 184–211). Washington, DC: American Psychiatric Press.

Layne, C. M., Pynoos, R. S., Saltzman, W. S., Arslanagic, B., Black, M., Savjak, N., et al. (2001). Trauma/grief-focused psychotherapy: School-based post-war intervention with traumatized Bosnian adolescents. *Group Dynamics: Theory, Research, and Practice, 5*(4), 277–290.

McLeer, S., Deblinger, E., Henry, D., & Orvaschel, H. (1992). Sexually abused children at high risk for post-traumatic stress disorder, *Journal of the American Academy of Child and Adolescent Psychiatry, 31*(5), 875–879.

Melhem, N. M., Day, N. Shear, M. K., Day, R., Reynolds, C. F., & Brent, D. (2004). Traumatic grief among adolescents exposed to a peer's suicide. *American Journal of Psychiatry, 161*(8), 1411–1416.

Moles, K. (2001). *The teen relationship workbook.* Plainview, NY: Wellness Reproductions and Publishing.

Nader, K. O. (1996). Children's exposure to traumatic experiences. In C. A. Corr & D. M. Corr (Eds.), *Handbook of childhood death and bereavement* (pp. 201–220). New York: Springer.

Nader, K. (1997) Childhood traumatic loss: The interaction of trauma and grief. In C. R. Figley, B. Bride, & N. Mazza (Eds.), *Death and trauma: The traumatology of grieving* (pp. 17–41). Washington, DC: Taylor & Francis.

Nemeroff, C. B., Heim, C. M. Thase, M. E., Klein, D. N., Rush, A. J., Schatzberg, A. F. et al. (2003). Differential responses to psychotherapy versus pharmacotherapy in patients with chronic forms of major depression and childhood trauma. *Proceedings of the National Academy of Sciences of the United States of America, 100*(24), 14293–14296.

Pfeffer, C. R., Jiang, H., Kakuma, T., Hwang, J., & Metsch, M. (2002). Group intervention for children bereaved by the suicide of a relative. *Journal of the American Academy of Child and Adolescent Psychiatry, 41*(5), 505–513.

Prigerson, H. G., & Jacobs, S. C. (2001). Diagnostic criteria for traumatic grief. In M. S. Stroebe, R. O. Hansson, W. Stroebe, & H. Schut (Eds.), *Handbook of bereavement research* (pp. 614–646). Washington DC: American Psychological Association.

Pynoos, R. (1992). Grief and trauma in children and adolescents. *Bereavement Care, 11*(1), 2–10.

Pynoos, R. S., Goenjian, A. K., & Steinberg, A. M. (1998). A public mental health approach to the postdisaster treatment of children and adolescents. *Child and Adolescent Psychiatric Clinics of North America, 7,* 195–210.

Pynoos, R., & Nader, K. (1990). Children's exposure to violence and traumatic death. *Psychiatric Annals, 20*(6), 334–344.

Raphael, B. (1997). The interaction of trauma and grief. In D. Black & M. Newman (Eds.), *Psychological trauma: A developmental approach* (pp. 31–43). Arlington, VA: American Psychiatric Press.

Raphael, B., Martinek, N., & Wooding, S. (2004). Assessing traumatic bereavement and posttraumatic stress disorder. In J. P. Wilson & T. M. Keane (Eds.), *Assessing psychological trauma and PTSD* (2nd ed., pp. 492–510). New York: Guilford Press.

Rodriguez, N., Steinberg, A. M., & Pynoos, R. S. (1999). *UCLA PTSD for DSM IV Index—Adolescent Version.* Unpublished manuscript, University of California at Los Angeles.

Saltzman, W. R., Pynoos, R. S., Layne, C. M., Steinberg, A. M., & Aisenberg, E. (2001). Trauma/grief focused intervention for adolescents exposed to community violence: Results of a school-based screening and group treatment protocol. *Group Dynamics: Theory, Research and Practice, 5*(4), 291–303.

Scheeringa, M. S., Peebles, C. D., Cook, C. A., & Zeanah, C. H. (2001). Toward establishing procedural criterion and discriminant validity for PTSD in early childhood. *Journal of the American Academy of Child and Adolescent Psychiatry, 40,* 52–60.

Scheeringa, M. S., Zeanah, C. H., Drell, M. J., & Larrieu, J. A. (1995). Two approaches to diagnosing PTSD in infancy and early childhood. *Journal of the American Academy of Child and Adolescent Psychiatry, 34,* 191–200.

Sigman, M., & Wilson, J. P. (1998). Traumatic bereavement: Post traumatic stress disorder and prolonged grief in motherless daughters. *Journal of Psychological Practice, 4*(1), 34–50.

Stein, N. L. (2002). Memories for emotional, stressful, and traumatic events. In N. L. Stein, P. J. Bauer, & M. Rabinowitz (Eds.), *Representation, memory, and development: Essays in honor of Jean Mandler* (pp. 247–265). Mahwah, NJ: Erlbaum.

Sternberg, K. J., Lamb, M. E., Hershkowitz, I., Yudilevitch, L. Orbach, Y., Esplin, P. W., et al. (1997). Effects of introductory style on children's abilities to describe experiences of sexual abuse. *Child Abuse and Neglect, 21*(11), 1133–1146.

Tagney, J. P. (1999). The self-conscious emotions: Shame, guilt, embarrassment and pride. In T. Dalgleish & M. Power (Eds.), *Handbook of cognition and emotion*. New York: Wiley.

Teichner, M. H. (2002, March). Scars that won't heal: The neurobiology of child abuse. *Scientific American*, 68–75.

Williams, M. B., & Poijula, S. (2002). *The PTSD workbook*. Oakland, CA: New Harbinger.

Wraith, R. (1997, May 7–10). Debriefing for children: What is it we should be thinking about? Traumatic grief-growing at different life stages. *Proceedings of the Joint National Conference of the National Association of Loss and Grief, Australasian Critical Incident Stress Association, and Australasian Society of Traumatic Stress Studies: Trauma, Grief and Growth— Finding a Path to Healing*, Sydney, Australia, 384–386.

GAMES

Black, C. (1984). *The Stamp Game: A game of feelings*. Denver: MAC Printing.

Burke, C. R. *Survivor's journey: A therapeutic game for working with survivor's of sexual abuse*. Available from www.creativetherapystore.com.

Cavanaugh-Johnson, T. *Let's talk about touching: A therapeutic game*. Available from Toni Cavanaugh Johnson, 1101 Fremont Avenue, Suite 101, South Pasadena, CA 91030.

Dlugokinski, E. *Dealing with feelings card game*. Available from www.creativetherapystore.com.

The Goodbye Game, M & B Distributors; PH: 1(204) 728-3758; www.childswork.com

The Grief Game, Jessica Kingsley Publishers, 116 Pentonville RD, London N1 9JB; www.jkp.com

The Mad, Sad, Glad Game (1990). Loveland, CO: Peak Potential.

Mitlin, M. *Emotional Bingo*. Available from www.creativetherapystore.com.

WEBSITES

American Professional Society on the Abuse of Children
www.apsac.org

CARES Institute
Child Abuse Research Education Service
School of Osteopathic Medicine
University of Medicine and Dentistry of New Jersey
www.caresinstitute.org

Center for Traumatic Stress in Children and Adolescents
Allegheny General Hospital
www.pittsburghchildtrauma.org

Creative Therapy Associates
www.ctherapy.com (*How Are You Feeling Today* posters and supplies).

International Society for Traumatic Stress Studies
www.istss.org

National Child Traumatic Stress Network
www.nctsnet.org

National Crime Victims Research and Treatment Center
Medical University of South Carolina
www.musc.edu/cvc

APPENDIX 3

ADDITIONAL TRAINING

TF-CBTWEB

TF-CBTWeb is a web-based training course for learning trauma-focused cognitive-behavioral therapy, sponsored by the Medical University of South Carolina. It covers all of the procedures of TF-CBT and includes streaming video demonstrations, clinical scripts, cultural considerations, clinical challenges, and many other learning resources.

TF-CBTWeb was developed for busy mental health professionals who want to learn the best evidence-based treatments, but who need a flexible, cost-effective, and convenient way of learning on their own schedule. Professionals who complete the full TF-CBTWeb course receive a Certificate of Completion for 10 continuing education contact hours. The Medical University of South Carolina is an approved provider of continuing education for all mental health professionals. TF-CBTWeb is free to all users. It is compatible with both PC and Macintosh computers, and with most major web browsers such as Internet Explorer, Firefox, Mozilla, and Netscape.

To learn more about TF-CBTWeb, go to www.musc.edu/tfcbt.

NATIONAL CHILD TRAUMATIC STRESS NETWORK

The Childhood Traumatic Grief Educational Materials are available on the NCTSN website and through the national resource center (for the duration of the NCTSN). These provide additional training to professionals in the CTG treatment model. In particular, "The Courage to Remember" video and accompanying print curriculum (which is available in print form and downloadable format on the website) provide information about our CTG treatment model. It is available at www.nctsnet.org. The NCTSN is funded by the Substance Abuse and Mental Health Services Administration (SAMHSA).

References

Achenbach, T. M. (1991). *Manual for the Child Behavior Checklist/4–18 and 1991 profile.* Burlington, VT: Department of Psychiatry, University of Vermont.

Ahmad, A., & Mohammad, K. (1996). The socioemotional development of orphans in orphanages and traditional foster care in Iraqi Kurdistan. *Child Abuse and Neglect, 20,* 1161–1173.

Alexander, D. W. (1993a). *All my dreams.* Creative Healing Book Series. Plainview, NY: Bureau for At-Risk Youth.

Alexander, D. W. (1993b). *It happened in autumn.* Creative Healing Book Series. Plainview, NY: Bureau for At-Risk Youth.

Alexander, D. W. (1993c). *It's my life.* Creative Healing Book Series. Plainview, NY: Bureau for At-Risk Youth.

Alexander, D. W. (1993d). *When I remember.* Creative Healing Book Series. Plainview, NY: Bureau for At-Risk Youth.

American Academy of Child and Adolescent Psychiatry. (1997). Practice parameters for the assessment and treatment of children and adolescents with substance use disorders. *Journal of the American Academy of Child and Adolescent Psychiatry, 36*(Suppl.), 140S–156S.

American Academy of Child and Adolescent Psychiatry. (1998). Practice parameters for the diagnosis and treatment of posttraumatic stress disorder in children and adolescents. *Journal of the American Academy of Child and Adolescent Psychiatry, 37*(10, Suppl.), 4S–26S.

American Psychiatric Association. (2000). *Diagnostic and statistical manual of mental disorders* (4th ed., text rev.). Washington, DC: Author.

Arata, C. M. (2000). From child victim to adult victim: A model for predicting sexual revictimization. *Child Maltreatment, 5,* 28–38.

Asmundson, G. J., Stapleton, J. A., & Taylor, S. (2004). Are avoidance and numbing distinct PTSD symptom clusters? *Journal of Traumatic Stress, 17,* 467–475.

Bancroft, L., & Silverman, J. G. (2002). *The batterer as parent.* Thousand Oaks, CA: Sage.

Barkley, R. (2000). *Taking charge of ADHD: The complete, authoritative guide for parents* (rev. ed.). New York: Guilford Press.

Beck, A. T., Steer, R. A., & Brown, G. K. (1996). *BDI-II: Beck Depression Inventory Manual* (2nd ed.). San Antonio, TX: Psychological Corporation.

Beck, J. S. (1995). *Cognitive therapy: Basics and beyond.* New York: Guilford Press.

Beck, J. S., Beck, A. T., & Jolly, J. B. (2001). *Beck Youth Depression Inventory.* San Antonio, TX: Psychological Corporation.

Benson, H. (1975). *The relaxation response.* New York: Avon Books.

Birmaher, B. (2004). *New hope for children and teens with bipolar disorder: Your friendly authoritative guide to the latest in traditional and complementary solutions.* New York: Three Rivers Press.

Birmaher, B., Khetarpal, S., Brent, D., Cully, M., Balach, L., Kaufman, J., et al. (1997). The Screen for Child Anxiety Related Emotional Disorders (SCARED): Scale construction and psychometric characteristics. *Journal of the American Academy of Child and Adolescent Psychiatry, 36,* 545–553.

Black, C. (1984). *The Stamp Game: A game of feelings.* Denver: MAC Printing.

Black, D. (1998). Coping with loss, bereavement in childhood. *British Medical Journal, 316,* 931–933.

Bloomquist, M. L. (2006). *Skills training for children with behavior problems (rev. ed.): A parent and therapist guidebook.* New York: Guilford Press.

Boney-McCoy, S., & Finkelhor, D. (1995). Prior victimization: A risk factor for child sexual abuse and for PTSD related symptomatology among sexually abused youth. *Child Abuse and Neglect, 19*(12), 1401–1421.

Briere, J. (1995). *Trauma Symptom Checklist for Children (TSC-C) Manual.* Odessa, FL: Psychological Assessment Resources.

Brown, E. J., Cohen, J. A., Amaya-Jackson, L., Handel, S., & Layne, C. (2003). *Characteristics and responses upon exposure to death (CARED youth report and CARED parent report).* New York: National Child Traumatic Stress Network, SAMHSA.

Brown, E. J., & Goodman, R. F. (2005). Childhood traumatic grief following September 11th, 2001: Construct development and validation. *Journal of Clinical Child and Adolescent Psychology, 34,* 248–259.

Brown, L. K., & Brown, M. (1996). *When dinosaurs die: A guide to understanding death.* Boston: Little, Brown.

Chemtob, C. M., Nakashima, J. P., & Hamada, R. S. (2002). Psychosocial interventions for postdisaster trauma symptoms in elementary school children. *Archives of Pediatric and Adolescent Medicine, 156,* 211–216.

Christ, G. H. (2000). *Healing children's grief: Surviving a parent's death from cancer.* New York: Oxford University Press.

Cloitre, M., Davis, L., & Mirvis, S. (2002). *A phase-based treatment for adolescent trauma survivors of childhood abuse.* Report to the DeWitt Wallace/New York Hospital Fund, New York.

Cohen, J. A., Deblinger, E., Mannarino, A. P., & De Arellano, M. A. (2001). The importance of culture in treating abused and neglected children: An empirical review. *Child Maltreatment, 6*(2), 148–157.

Cohen, J. A., Deblinger, E., Mannarino, A. P., & Steer, R. A. (2004). A multisite, randomized controlled trial for children with sexual abuse-related PTSD symptoms. *Journal of the American Academy of Child and Adolescent Psychiatry, 43,* 393–402.

Cohen, J. A., Greenberg, T., Padlo, S., Shipley, C., Mannarino, A. P., Deblinger, E., et al. (2001). *Cognitive behavioral therapy for traumatic grief in children.* Unpublished treatment manual, Allegheny General Hospital, Pittsburgh, PA.

Cohen, J. A., & Mannarino, A. P. (1992). *Trauma-focused CBT for sexually abused preschool children.* Unpublished treatment manual, University of Pittsburgh School of Medicine, Pittsburgh, PA.

Cohen, J. A., & Mannarino, A. P. (1993). A treatment model for sexually abused preschoolers. *Journal of Interpersonal Violence, 8*(1), 115–131.

Cohen, J. A., & Mannarino, A. P. (1994). *Trauma-focused CBT treatment manual for children and adolescents.* Unpublished treatment manual, MCP-Hahnemann University School of Medicine, Allegheny General Hospital, Pittsburgh, PA.

Cohen, J. A., & Mannarino, A. P. (1996a). A treatment outcome study for sexually abused preschooler children: Initial findings. *Journal of the American Academy of Child and Adolescent Psychiatry, 35*(1), 42–50.

Cohen, J. A., & Mannarino, A. P. (1996b). Factors that mediate treatment outcome of sexually abused preschool children. *Journal of the American Academy of Child and Adolescent Psychiatry, 35*(10), 1402–1410.

Cohen, J. A., & Mannarino, A. P. (1998a). Interventions for sexually abused children: Initial treatment findings. *Child Maltreatment, 3*(1), 17–26.

Cohen, J. A., & Mannarino, A. P. (1998b). Factors that mediate treatment outcome of sexually abused preschoolers: Six and 12-month follow-ups. *Journal of the American Academy of Child and Adolescent Psychiatry, 37,* 44–51.

Cohen, J. A., & Mannarino, A. P. (2000). Predictors of treatment outcome in sexually abused children. *Child Abuse and Neglect, 24*(7), 983–994.

Cohen, J. A., Mannarino, A. P., & Knudsen, K. (2004). Treating childhood traumatic grief: A pilot study. *Journal of the American Academy of Child and Adolescent Psychiatry, 43,* 1225–1233.

Cohen, J. A., Mannarino, A. P., & Staron, V. (2005). *A pilot study of modified cognitive behavioral therapy for children with traumatic grief.* Manuscript in review.

Cunningham, C. (1992). *All kinds of separation.* Indianapolis: Kidsrights.

Davis, M., Eshelman, E. R., & McKay, M. (1988). *The relaxation and stress reduction workbook* (3rd ed.). Oakland, CA: New Harbinger.

De Bellis, M. D., Baum, A. S., Birmaher, B., Keshavan, M. S., Eccard, C. H., Boring, A. M., et al. (1999). Developmental traumatology: Part I. Biological stress systems. *Biological Psychiatry, 45,* 1259–1270.

De Bellis, M. D., Keshavan, M. S., Clark, D. B., Casey, B. J., Giedd, J. N., Boring, A. M., et al. (1999). Developmental traumatology: Part II. Brain development. *Biological Psychiatry, 45,* 1271–1284.

Deblinger, E., Behl, L. E., & Glickman, A. R. (2006). Treating children who have experienced sexual abuse. In P. C. Kendall (Ed.), *Child and adolescent therapy: Cognitive-behavioral procedures* (3rd ed., pp. 383–416). New York: Guilford Press.

Deblinger, E., & Heflin, A. H. (1996). *Treating sexually abused children and their nonoffending parents: A cognitive behavioral approach.* Thousand Oaks, CA: Sage.

Deblinger, E., Lippmann, J., & Steer, R. (1996). Sexually abused children suffering posttraumatic stress symptoms: Initial treatment outcome findings. *Child Maltreatment, 1*(4), 310–321.

Deblinger, E., Mannarino, A. P., Cohen, J. A., & Steer, R. (2005). *A multisite, randomized controlled trial for children with sexual abuse-related PTSD symptoms: A follow-up and examination of predictors of treatment response.* Manuscript submitted for publication.

Deblinger, F., McLeer, S. V., Atkins, M., Ralphe, D., & Foa, E. (1989). Posttraumatic stress in sexually abused, physically abused and nonabused children. *Child Abuse and Neglect, 13*, 403–408.

Deblinger, E., McLeer, S. V., & Henry, D. (1990). Cognitive-behavioral treatment for sexually abused children suffering post-traumatic stress: Preliminary findings. *Journal of the American Academy of Child and Adolescent Psychiatry, 29*, 747–752.

Deblinger, E., Stauffer, L. B., & Steer, R. (2001). Comparative efficacies of supportive and cognitive-behavioral group therapies for young children who have been sexually abused and their non-offending mothers. *Child Maltreatment, 6*, 332–343.

Deblinger, E., Steer, B., & Lippmann, J. (1999). Maternal factors associated with sexually abused children's psychosocial adjustment. *Child Maltreatment, 4*, 13–20.

Derogatis, L. R., Lipman, R. S., & Covi, L. (1973). SCL-90: An outpatient psychiatric rating scale—preliminary report. *Psychopharmacology Bulletin, 9*(1), 13–28.

DeRosa, R. (2004). *Structured Psychotherapy for Adolescents Responding to Chronic Stress (SPARCS).* Manhasset, NY: Unpublished treatment manual.

DiNicola, V. F. (1996). Ethnocentric aspects of PTSD and related disorders among children and adolescents. In A. J. Marsalla, M. J. Friedman, E. T. Gerrity, & R. M. Scurfield (Eds.), *Ethnocultural aspects of PTSD: Issues, research and clinical applications* (pp. 389–414). Washington, DC: American Psychological Association.

Eth, S., & Pynoos, R. S. (1985). Interaction of trauma and grief in childhood. In S. Eth & R. S. Pynoos (Eds.), *Posttraumatic stress disorder in children* (pp. 171–186). Washington, DC: American Psychiatric Association.

Feiring, C., Taska, L., & Lewis, M. (2002). Adjustment following sexual abuse discovery: The role of shame and attributional style. *Developmental Psychology, 38*, 79–92.

Finkelhor, D., Asdigian, N., & Dzuiba-Leatherman, J. (1995). The effectiveness of victimization prevention instruction: An evaluation of children's responses to actual threats and assaults. *Child Abuse and Neglect, 19*(2), 141–153

Fitzgerald, H. (1992). *The grieving child: A parent's guide.* New York: Simon & Schuster.

Fitzgerald, H. (1995). *The mourning handbook: The most comprehensive resource offering practical and compassionate advice on coping with all aspects of death and dying.* New York: Simon & Schuster.

Foa, E. B., Molnar, C., & Cashman, L. (1995). Change in rape narratives during exposure therapy for PTSD. *Journal of Traumatic Stress, 8*, 675–690.

Ford, J. D., Racusin, R., Daviss, W. B., Ellis, C. G., Thomas, J., Rogers, K., et al. (1999). Trauma exposure among children with oppositional defiant disorder and attention deficit-hyperactivity disorder. *Journal of Consulting and Clinical Psychiatry, 67*(5), 786–789.

Fox, S. S. (1985). *Good grief: Helping groups of children when a friend dies.* Boston: New England Association for the Education of Young Children.

Frankl, V. E. (1985). Paradoxical intention. In G. R. Weeks (Ed.), *Promoting change through paradoxical therapy*. Homewood, IL: Dow Jones-Irwin.

Gidron, Y., Peri, T., Connolly, J. F., & Shalev, A. Y. (1996). Written disclosure in PTSD: Is it beneficial for the patient? *Journal of Nervous and Mental Disease, 185*, 505–507.

Goenjian, A. K., Karaya, I., Pynoos, R. S., Minassian, D., Najarian, L. M., Steinberg, A. M., et al. (1997). Outcome of psychotherapy among early adolescents after trauma. *American Journal of Psychiatry, 154*, 536–542.

Goldman, L. (1996). *Breaking the silence: A guide to help children with complicated grief—suicide, homicide, AIDS, violence and abuse*. London: Taylor & Francis.

Goldman, L. (1998). *Bart speaks out: Breaking the silence on suicide*. Los Angeles: Manson Western Corporation.

Goldman, L. (2000). *Life and loss: A guide to help grieving children* (2nd ed.). London: Taylor & Francis.

Harrington, R., & Harrison, L. (1999). Unproven assumptions about the impact of bereavement on children. *Journal of the Royal Society of Medicine, 92*, 230–233.

Harris, R. H. (2001). *Good-bye mousie*. New York: Margaret K. McElderry Books.

Hemery, K. (1998). *The brightest star*. Omaha, NE: Centering Corporation.

Holmes, M. M. (1999a). *Molly's mom died: A child's book of hope through grief*. Omaha, NE: Centering Corporation.

Holmes, M. M. (1999b). *Sam's dad died: A child's book of hope through grief*. Omaha, NE: Centering Corporation.

Holmes, M. M. (2000). *A terrible thing happened*. Washington, DC: Magination Press.

Jacobs, S. (1999). *Traumatic grief: Diagnosis, treatment and prevention*. Philadelphia: Brunner/Mazel.

Jenkins, E. J., & Bell, C. C. (1994). Exposure to violence, psychological distress, and risk behaviors in a sample of inner city high school students. In S. Friedman (Ed.), *Anxiety disorders in African Americans* (pp. 76–88). New York: Springer.

Jessie. (1991). *Please tell*. Center City, MN: Hazelden Foundation.

Joseph, S. A., Williams, R., Yule, W., & Walker, A. (1992). Factor analysis of the Impact of Events Scale with survivors of two disasters at sea. *Personality and Individual Differences, 13*, 693–697.

Kabat-Zinn, J. (1990). *Full catastrophe living: Using the wisdom of your body and mind to face stress, pain, and illness*. New York: Delta.

Kataoka, S. H., Stein, B. D., Jaycox, L. H., Wong, M., Escudero, P., Windl, T., et al. (2003). A school-based mental health program for traumatized Latino immigrant children. *Journal of the American Academy of Child and Adolescent Psychiatry, 42*, 311–318.

King, N. J., Tonge, B. J., Mullen, P., Myerson, N., Heyne, D., Rollings, S., et al. (2000). Treating sexually abused children with posttraumatic stress symptoms: A randomized clinical trial. *Journal of the American Academy of Child and Adolescent Psychiatry, 39*, 1347–1355.

Klein, I., & Janoff-Bulman, R. (1996). Trauma history and personal narratives: Some clues to coping among survivors of child abuse. *Child Abuse and Neglect, 20*, 45–54.

Kliewer, W., Murrelle, L., Mejia, R., Torresde, G. Y., & Angold, A. (2001). Exposure to violence against a family member and internalizing symptoms in Colombian adolescents: The protective effects of family support. *Journal of Consulting and Clinical Psychology, 69,* 971–982.

Kolko, D. J. (1996). Individual cognitive behavioral treatment and family therapy for physically abused children and their offending parents: A comparison of clinical outcomes. *Child Maltreatment, 1,* 322–342.

Kolko, D. J., & Swenson, C. C. (2002). *Assessing and treating physically abused children and their families: A cognitive behavioral approach.* Thousand Oaks, CA: Sage.

Kovacs, M. (1985). The Children's Depression Inventory (CDI). *Psychopharmacology Bulletin, 113,* 164–180.

LaGreca, A. M., Silverman, W. K., & Wasserstein, S. B. (1998). Children's predisaster functioning as a predictor of posttraumatic stress following Hurricane Andrew. *Journal of Consulting and Clinical Psychology, 66,* 883–892.

Lamb-Shapiro, J. (2000). *The hyena who lost her laugh: A story about changing your negative thinking.* Plainview, NY: Childswork/Childsplay.

Laor, N., Wolmer, L., & Cohen, D. J. (2001). Mothers' functioning and children's symptoms five years after a SCUD missile attack. *American Journal of Psychiatry, 158,* 1020–1026.

Layne, C. M., Pynoos, R. S., Saltzman, W. R., Arslanagic, B., Black, M., & Savjak, N., et al. (2001). Trauma/grief-focused group psychotherapy: School based post-war intervention with traumatized Bosnian adolescents. *Group Dynamics: Theory, Research and Practice, 5*(4), 277–290.

Layne, C. M., Saltzman, W. S., Savjak, N., & Pynoos, R. S. (1999). *Trauma/grief-focused group psychotherapy manual.* Sarajevo, Bosnia: UNICEF Bosnia & Herzegovina.

Layne, C. M., Savjak, N., Saltzman, W. R., & Pynoos, R. S. (2001). *UCLA/BYU Expanded Grief Inventory.* Unpublished instrument, Brigham Young University, Provo, UT (Available from the first author at Christopher. layne@byu.edu).

Mad Sad Glad Game. (1990). Loveland, CO: Peak Potential.

Mannarino, A. P., & Cohen, J. A. (1996). Family related variable and psychological symptom formation in sexually abused girls. *Journal of Child Sexual Abuse, 5,* 105–119.

Mannarino, A. P., Cohen, J. A., & Berman, S. (1994). The Children's Attribution and Perceptions Scale: Methodological implications of a two-stage survey. *Child Abuse and Neglect, 16,* 399–407.

March, J. S., Amaya-Jackson, L., Murray M. C., & Schulte, A. (1998). Cognitive-behavioral psychotherapy for children and adolescents with PTSD after a single-episode stressor. *Journal of the American Academy of Child and Adolescent Psychiatry, 37,* 585–593.

March, J. S., Parker, J. D. A., Sullivan, K., Stallings, P., & Conners, C. K. (1997). The Multidimensional Anxiety Scale for Children: Factor structure, reliability and validity. *Journal of the American Academy of Child and Adolescent Psychiatry, 36*(4), 554–565.

Melham, N. M., Day, N., Shear, M. K., Day, R., Reynolds, C. F., & Brent, D. (2004). Traumatic grief among adolescents exposed to a peer's suicide. *American Journal of Psychiatry, 161,* 1411–1416.

Mitlin, M. (1998). *Emotional bingo: Creative therapy store.* Los Angeles: WPS Publishers.

Mueser, K. T., Jankowski, M. K., Rosenberg, H. J., Rosenberg, S. D., & Hamblen, J. L. (2004). *Cognitive-behavioral therapy for PTSD in adolescents [provider manual]*. Lebanon, NH: Dartmouth Medical School and New Hampshire–Dartmouth Psychiatric Research Center.

Nader, K. O. (1997). Childhood traumatic loss: The interaction of trauma and grief. In C. R. Figley, B. E. Bride, & N. Mazza (Eds.), *Death and trauma: The traumatology of grieving* (pp. 17–41). New York: Hamilton Printing.

Najavits, L. M. (1998). *Cognitive-behavioral therapy for PTSD/alcohol use disorder in adolescent girls* (NIAAA Grant No. R21 AA12818), MacLean Hospital, Belmont, MA.

Najavits, L. M. (2002). *Seeking safety: A treatment manual for PTSD and substance abuse*. New York: Guilford Press.

O'Connor, K. J. (1983). Color Your Life technique. In C. E. Schaefer & K. J. O'Connor (Eds.), *Handbook of play therapy* (pp. 251–258). New York: Wiley.

Pennebaker, J. W. (1993). Putting stress into words: Health, linguistic and therapeutic implications. *Behavioral Research Therapy, 31,* 539–548.

Pennebaker, J. W., & Francis, M. (1996). Cognitive, emotional and language processes in disclosure. *Cognitions and Emotion, 10,* 601–626.

Pine, D. S., & Cohen, J. A. (2002). Trauma in children: Risk and treatment of psychiatric sequelae. *Biological Psychiatry, 51,* 519–531.

Pine, D. S., Mogg, K., Bradley, B., Montgomery, L. A., Monk, C. S., McClure E., et al. (2005). Attention bias to threat in maltreated children: Implications for vulnerability to stress-related psychopathology. *American Journal of Psychiatry, 162,* 291–296.

Prigerson, H. G., & Jacobs, S. C. (2001). Caring for bereaved patients: All the doctors just suddenly go. *Journal of the American Medical Association, 286*(11), 1369–1376.

Prigerson, H. G., Maciejewski, P. K., Reynolds, C. F., Bierhals, A. J., Newsom, J. T., Fisiczka, A., et al. (1995). Inventory of Complicated Grief: A scale to measure maladaptive symptoms of loss. *Psychiatric Research, 59,* 65–79.

Prigerson, H. G., Shear, M. K., Frank, E., Beery, L. C., Silberman, R., Prigerson, J., et al. (1997). Traumatic grief: A case of loss-induced trauma. *American Journal of Psychiatry, 154*(7), 1003–1009.

Prigerson, H. G., Shear, M. K., & Jacobs, S. C. (1999). Concensus criteria for traumatic grief: A preliminary empirical test. *British Journal of Psychiatry, 174,* 67–73.

Putnam, F. W. (2003). Ten year research update review: Child sexual abuse. *Journal of the American Academy of Child and Adolescent Psychiatry, 42,* 269–278.

Pynoos, R. S. (1992). Grief and trauma in children and adolescents. *Bereavement Care, 11,* 2–10.

Pynoos, R. S., & Nader, K. (1988). Psychological first aid and treatment approach for children exposed to community violence: Research implications. *Journal of Traumatic Stress, 1,* 445–473.

Pynoos, R. S., Rodriguez, N., Steinberg, A., Stuber, M., & Fredrick, C. (1998). *The UCLA PTSD Index for DSM-IV, Parent Version*. Unpublished psychological instrument (Available from the National Child Traumatic Stress Network website, www.nctsnet.org).

Rando, T. A. (1993). *Treatment of complicated mourning*. Ottawa, ON: Research Press.

Rando, T. A. (1996). Complications of mourning traumatic death. In K. J. Dolca (Ed.), *Living with grief after sudden loss*. Washington, DC: Hospice Foundation of America.

Rey, J. M., Schrader, E., & Morris-Yates, A. (1992). Parent–child agreement on children's behaviors reported by the Child Behavior Checklist (CBCL). *Journal of Adolescence, 15*, 219–230.

Reynolds, C. R., & Kamphaus, R. W. (1992). *Behavioral Assessment System for Children Manual*. Circle Pines, MN: American Guidance Service.

Riverdeep Interactive Learning Limited. (2005). *Storybook Weaver*. San Francisco: Riverdeep Interactive Learning Limited.

Romain, T. (1999). *What on earth do you do when someone dies?* Minneapolis, MN: Free Spirit Publishing.

Runyon, M., Basilio, I., Van Hasselt, V. B., & Hersen, M. (1998). Child witnesses of interparental violence: A manual for child and family treatment. In V. B. Van Hasselt & M. Hersen (Eds.), *Sourcebook of psychological treatment manuals for children and adolescents* (pp. 203–278). Hillsdale, NJ: Erlbaum.

Ryan, G. (1989). Victim to victimizer: Rethinking victim treatment. *Journal of Interpersonal Violence, 4*(3), 325–341.

Saunders, B. E. (2003). Understanding children exposed to violence: Toward an integration of overlapping fields. *Journal of Interpersonal Violence, 18*, 356–376.

Saunders, B. E., Berliner, L., & Hanson, R. F. (Eds.). (2001, April 26). *Child physical and sexual abuse: Guidelines for treatment* (Revised report). Charleston, SC: National Crime Victims Research and Treatment Center.

Scheeringa, M. S., Zeanah, C. H., Myers, L., & Putnam, F. W. (2003). New findings on alternative criteria for PTSD in preschool children. *Journal of the American Academy of Child and Adolescent Psychiatry, 42*(5), 561–570.

Schor, H. (2002). *A place for Starr: A story of hope for children experiencing family violence*. Indianapolis: Kidsrights.

Seligman, M. E. P. (1998). *Learned optimism: How to change your mind and your life* (2nd ed.). New York: Knopf.

Seligman, M., Reivich, K., Jaycox, L., & Gillham, J. (1995). *The optimistic child*. New York: Houghton Mifflin.

Sheppard, C. H. (1996). *Brave Bart: A story for traumatized and grieving children*. Grosse Pointe Woods, MI: Institute for Trauma and Loss in Children.

Siegel, K., Karus, D., & Raveis, V. (1996). Adjustment of children facing death of a parent due to cancer. *Journal of the American Academy of Child and Adolescent Psychiatry, 35*(4), 442–450.

Siegel, K., Raveis, V., & Karus, D. (1996). Patterns of communication with children when a parent has cancer. In C. Cooper, L. Baider, & A. Kaplan DeNour (Eds.), *Cancer and the family* (pp. 109–128). New York: Wiley.

Simpson, M. A. (1997). Traumatic bereavements and death-related PTSD. In C. R. Figley, B. E. Bride, & N. Mazza (Eds.), *Death and trauma: The traumatology of grieving* (pp. 3–16). Washington, DC: Taylor & Francis.

Spaccareli, S. (1994). Stress, appraisal, and coping in child sexual abuse: A theoretical and empirical review. *Psychological Bulletin, 116*, 340–362.

Spielberger, C. D. (1973). *Manual for the State–Trait Anxiety Inventory for Children*. Palo Alto, CA: Consulting Psychologists Press.

Stauffer, L., & Deblinger, E. (1996). Cognitive behavioral groups for non-offending

mothers and their young sexually abused children: A preliminary treatment outcome study. *Child Maltreatment, 1,* 65–76.

Stauffer, L. B., & Deblinger, E. (2003). *Let's talk about taking care of you: An educational book about body safety.* Hatfield, PA: Hope for Families.

Stauffer, L. B., & Deblinger, E. (2004). *Let's talk about taking care of you: An educational book about body safety for young children.* Hatfield, PA: Hope for Families.

Stein, B. D., Jaycox, L. H., Kataoka, S. H., Wong, M., Tu, W., Elliott, M. N., et al.
(2003). A mental health intervention for school children exposed to violence: A
randomized controlled trial. *Journal of the American Medical Association, 290,*
603–611.

Sternberg, K. J., Lamb, M. E., Hershkowitz, I., Yudilevitch, L., Orbach, Y., Esplin, P.
W., et al. (1997). Effects of introductory style on children's abilities to describe
experiences of sexual abuse. *Child Abuse and Neglect, 21,* 1133–1146.

Stubenbort, K., Donnelly, G. R., & Cohen, J. (2001). Cognitive-behavioral group
therapy for bereaved adults and children following an air disaster. *Group
Dynamics: Theory, Research and Practice, 5,* 261–276.

Thomas, P. (2001). *I miss you: A first look at death.* Hauppauge, NY: Barrons.

Webb, N. B. (1993). *Helping bereaved children.* New York: Guilford Press.

Webb, N. B. (2002). Traumatic death of a friend/peer: Case of Susan, age 9. In N. B.
Webb (Ed.), *Helping bereaved children* (2nd ed., pp. 167–194). New York:
Guilford Press.

Wolfe, V. V., Gentile, C., Michienzi, T., Sas, L., & Wolfe, D. A. (1991). The
Children's Impact of Events Scale: A measure of post-sexual abuse PTSD symptoms. *Behavioral Assessment, 13,* 159–183.

Wolfelt, A. (1991). Children. *Bereavement Magazine, 5*(1), 38–39.

Worden, J. W. (1996). *Children and grief: When a parent dies.* New York: Guilford
Press.

Index